Keto diet cookbook 2020

Tasty recipes to regain your best shape (including a 30day example recipes to burn fat)

[Dr Steven Green]

Upon using the contents and information contained in this book, you agree to hold harmless the Author from and against any damages, costs, and expenses, including any legal fees potentially resulting from the application of any of the information provided by this book. This disclaimer applies to any loss, damages or injury caused by the use and application, whether directly or indirectly, of any advice or information presented, whether for breach of contract, tort, negligence, personal injury, criminal intent, or under any other cause of action.

You agree to accept all risks of using the information presented inside this book.

You agree that by continuing to read this book, where appropriate and/or necessary, you shall consult a professional (including but not limited to your doctor, attorney, or financial advisor or such other advisor as needed) before using any of the suggested remedies, techniques, or information in this book.

Table of Contents

CHAPTER 10: SOUP RECIPES   100

CHAPTER 11: SNACKS RECIPES   120

CHAPTER 12: DINNER RECIPES — 136

INTRODUCTION

One of the biggest problems that most people face when seeking information about the Ketogenic diet is getting information that is reliable, accurate, and well-explained. It is difficult to find a book that explains to you the basics of a Ketogenic diet without leaving gaps in the information provided. This is why most people are confused by the Ketogenic diet and end up believing all the negative misconceptions about it.

That is where this book draws the line. This book focuses on explaining the key concepts that you need to know to get started on a Ketogenic diet. A lot of care has been taken to make sure that every topic is covered as extensively as possible without being too technical for the reader to understand. The language has been simplified and complex theories have been broken down in a clear manner.

I have taken the time to provide technical and scientific evidence to back up many of the concepts presented here. You will find links that will lead you to studies conducted by qualified researchers who have studied the Ketogenic diet for decades. These are not my personal opinions that you have been presented here. This is credible content that is backed by science.

Chapter 1: What is Ketogenic Diet?

To put it in simple terms, it's a high fat, low carb diet that can transform your body into a fat-burning device. One of the biggest strength of this regime, lyes in his simplicity. Ketogenic diets provide an appropriate amount of protein intake, an elevated level of fat, and a small intake of carbohydrates. It was developed in the first place as a different diet to control the signs of epilepsy in children. Daily meals give sufficient protein to ensure growth and repair under this regime. The calories are measured and provided in enough quantities to maintain the right weight and height for the child.

The keto diet transforms how your body metabolizes food into energy. Naturally, your body converts carbohydrates (imagine pasta and bread) into energy glucose. Eating lots of fat and few carbs bring you in ketosis, a metabolic condition where your body releases fat rather than carbs for fuel.

HISTORY OF KETOGENIC DIET

First, in 1924, at the Mayo Clinic, the ketogenic diet was instituted.

Dr. Russel Wilder found that the symptoms became less prevalent when epileptic patients were placed on a keto diet.

The classic diet contains a 4:1 fat-to-protein-carbohydrate ratio. Food sources of high carbohydrates are removed from the diet. High-carbohydrate products include fruits, starchy vegetables, pasta, grains, and sugar. In the decades since the introduction of antiepileptic drugs, the prominence of this diet as a means of epilepsy control decreased. It was easier for most patients and care providers to use pills than to follow the stringent ketogenic diet. Though, there are still a few, like Johns Hopkins Medical and several other medical facilities, who offer and use this regime as a therapy alternative. The interest in the ketogenic diet as a management alternative for epilepsy was revived during the mid-1990.

Jim Abrahams, a film producer, had a son who was two years old and who suffered from a seizure disorder. The child was treated with the ketogenic diet. After adherence to this regime, the seizures were adequately controlled. The family founded the Charlie Foundation because of its success. It contributed to the creation of ketogenic diet research. In 1997, First Do No Harm, a television show, helped to make this diet known to the public as a way of treatment. Ever since that, the scientific focus has been renewed on how the diet and its prospective other use can be improved.

THE CONCEPTS OF KETOGENIC DIET

The consumption of carbohydrates is reduced to 20-50 g / day.

The intake of protein is moderate.

Everything is based on sex, height, and other functions.

Calories dependent on fat consumption are balanced.

The distribution of calories typically follows:

- 70%-75% from fat

- 20-25% from sources of protein

- 5-10% from carbohydrates

The diet proportion is meant to induce and sustain ketosis.

WHY MORE FAT AND MODERATE PROTEINS?

Insulin and blood sugar levels are not affected by fats.

If used in large quantities, proteins can influence insulin and blood sugar. The ketogenic diet is therefore recommended for moderate consumption.

Approximately 56% of the excess protein consumed is turned into sugar. This overcomes the ketosis of fat-burning as the body reacts to the glucose released from the breakdown of proteins.

Lean proteins and insufficient dietary fats can lead to rabbit hunger. Rabbit hunger refers to the condition in which adequate fats are not present. That is particularly apparent in a diet mainly made up of lean proteins. Diarrhea is the principal symptom which can become severe and cause death. Diarrhea takes place in the first three days to a week of a pure lean protein diet. If, in the coming days, sufficient fats are not integrated, diarrhea will worsen, and dehydration and death may occur.

A heavy-fat diet could be safer depending on the fat type and source.

In addition to keeping carbohydrate consumption low, clean saturated fats in the diet improve the fat profile of your body. This diet increases the levels of HDL and reduces triglycerides. This kind of fat profile is associated with increased protection from cardiovascular problems and heart attacks.

HOW DOES THE DIET WORKS?

The ketogenic diet pushes the body into a stage of ketosis. The body tends primarily to use carbohydrates as energy sources. The reason is that carbohydrates can be easily digested and absorbed. When the body is without carbohydrates, fats and proteins are used. Essentially, the body uses energy in a hierarchical manner. First, while it is available, the body uses carbohydrates. As a next alternative source, the body moves into fats. The last stage, usually in extreme deprivation of carbohydrates and fat stores, is protein conversion into energy. The digestion of proteins leads to loss of muscle, as the body digests the muscle proteins. Generally, the body enters the process of ketosis during the fasting period. One example of this is during sleep. When the body rebuilds and expands through sleep, it continues to burn fats for energy. Carbohydrates constitute most calories in an ordinary average meal. The body carbohydrates are used as energy, while other nutrients (i.e., fats and proteins) are stored. Many calories in the ketogenic diet are composed of fats instead of carbohydrates. In a ketogenic diet, carbohydrate is minimal and is used instantly.

There is a distinct energy deficit due to the low intake of carbohydrates. The body turns the fats it has accumulated; that switches to a fat burner from a carbohydrate user. The fats in the recently consumed meal are not immediately used, instead, they are stored for future necessity. The fats that were already present in the organism, instead, are used as energy sources, while some are still preserved. Therefore, in order to provide the immediate energy required, the Ketogenic diet must have a high fat intake and yet have a portion to stock. Stored fat is extremely important so that the body does not absorb the protein in the muscles at fasting times. In addition, these cycles are standard in a series of days. Fasting periods occur in between meals and sleep. During these times, the body also needs a constant energy supply. Protein in the muscles is next in line as the source of energy if no stored fat is present; your regime needs to be high in fat in order to prevent this. Ketogenic diets are mainly designed to imitate starvation mode. This decreases calories and significantly eliminates carbohydrates, thus depriving the body of carbohydrates instantly and quickly convert the remains. That compels the body to shift to the mode in which consumes fat. It also induces the secretion of catecholamines (fat mobilizing hormones), cortisol (break-down and metabolic hormones), and growth hormones. This triad of hormones triggers the state of ketosis or a fat burn.

Chapter 2: Steps to Keto Success

Calculate and track your macros. Macronutrients (macros) are carbohydrates, fats, and proteins. An average person would need more fat and fewer carbs, while a professional athlete may need more protein and high carbohydrate consumption.

Track your calorie consumption. Skipping a meal here or there isn't harmful when it's occasional but restricting calories for longer periods can have negative effects on your health. Carb cycling also involves calorie cycling so you can switch from low-calorie to higher-calorie periods.

Keep an eye on the amount of cholesterol. If your cholesterol level is high, avoid saturated fats (found primarily in red meat) and opt for monounsaturated fats. Trans fats such as partially hydrogenated vegetable oils are out of the question; they can be found in margarine and other spreads, fried foods, packaged foods, and fast foods. On the other hand, you should increase soluble fiber, foods rich in omega-3 fatty acid (herring, salmon, mackerel, flaxseeds, and walnuts).

Replenish electrolytes. Just make sure that you are eating foods that contain electrolytes such as bouillon, leafy green, avocado, and Himalayan salt. Taking magnesium supplements may be beneficial on a keto diet.

A few more tips. Consume at least 8 glasses of water per day to stay hydrated on the ketogenic diet. Further, get regular exercise. It doesn't have to be anything special and time-consuming. Simply find an activity that fits into your schedule like walking, cycling, or stair climbing. Keep it simple since the ketogenic diet requires a little pre-planning. Stick to real and nutrient-dense foods and find good alternatives for your favorite carbs. I am sure you will find inspiration and motivation in these six hundred recipes. You will learn how to prepare keto pancakes, granola, desserts, waffles and snacks. It is all about variety and smart food choices, not rigid rules and restrictive diet plans. And remember – you are beautiful just the way you are, take a deep breath and love yourself.

Weigh Your Food: Being accurate about your macros is very crucial to the success of the ketogenic diet.

Make sure that invest in a good food scale so that you can monitor your macro intake. So, avoid the guesswork and use a scale to measure your food. If you have more money to spare, buy scales that you can connect to apps and websites.

- **Drink Water:** Staying hydrated is one of the most important rules when it comes to following any kinds of diet regimen. Start your day by consuming at least 8 to 16 ounces of water to allow the body to begin its natural cycle.

- **Exercise:** Remember that diet alone will not help you lose as much weight as you want. You can also do resistant training because it requires more protein to aid in muscle gain. This exercise is great for keeping your protein in check especially if you consumed more of it than fats. Make sure that you match this diet regimen with a high interval and high-intensity workout to improve your blood glucose levels. Exercise at least 25 minutes every day to see the best results.

• **Reduce Your Stress:** Stress can affect your hormone levels by causing your blood sugar level to rise thus increasing your cravings. Have you ever noticed why you often crave for sweets when you are stressed out? That's your hormone talking. While you cannot control the stress that comes your way, find ways on how to mitigate it. You can practice yoga, mindfulness, and breathing exercises to take away your stress.

• **Choose Quality Carbs:** Some of you may say that carb is carb no matter what form they exist in. But remember that not all carbs are created equally. There are carbs that are nutrient-rich and are found in non-starchy vegetables and some fruits. So, when making a meal plan, make sure that you use good quality carbs.

• **Stay Away from Diet Soda:** Just because it comes with the word "diet" with it does not mean that it is good for you. Diet soda uses a wide variety of sugar substitutes that tells your body that is has an overload of sugar thereby shutting the metabolism down. So, if you need to quench your thirst, drink sparkling water instead.

- **Get Enough Sleep:** Sleep is necessary in order for you to lose weight fast. Remember that the lack of sleep causes stress to the body. Stress, as I have discussed earlier can affect the hormone levels in your body thus increasing your cravings to constantly snack on food. So, make sure that you get at least 6 to 8 hours of sleep daily.

- **Intermittent Fasting:** If you truly want to lose weight fast with the ketogenic diet, you might want to consider pairing it with intermittent fasting. Intermittent fasting is when you fast for more than 12 hours so that your body will use up the stored fats as its primary fuel. Consume your keto-friendly meals within a short eating window time and the rest of the day should be dedicated to no food consumption so that your body can undergo the state of ketosis faster. For instance, you can go fasting from 2:00 pm to 8:00 am the following day. From 8:01 am to 1:59 pm, that is the only time you allow yourself to eat your meals.

Chapter 3: What to Eat and What to Avoid

What to Eat on Keto

Ketones form when a person follows a low carb/high protein diet. Once the body enters Ketosis, the liver uses the fat to produce the Ketones. The production of Ketones helps improve blood flow to the brain resulting in quicker thinking and improved concentration. This makes the Keto diet great for women who are struggling with brain fog during menopause and post menopause.

The Keto diet suggests typically a limit of 20 to 50 grams of carbohydrates per day. While this can seem like a challenge, there are so many other food alternatives. Eating Keto-friendly meals never have to be boring or bland.

Seafood

Shellfish and fish are fantastic Keto diet options, they're extremely low carb and fully of healthy vitamins.

Salmon and other types of fish are very high in B vitamins, selenium, and potassium.

You'll still want to make sure that you're checking the nutritional information to ensure your carb intake doesn't go over the recommended amount.

Here is a list of seafood and the carb content based on a weight of 3.5 ounces.

- Mussels — 7 grams

- Clams — 5 grams

- Oysters — 4 grams

- Octopus — 4 grams

- Squid — 3 grams

Sardines, salmon, mackerel, and other types of fatty fish are incredibly high in omega-3, which has been found to lower the insulin levels, as well as increase sensitivity to insulin in those who are obese. Also, frequently eating fish has also been linked to improving mental health, including depression and mood swings.

We suggest eating two servings of seafood weekly while on your Keto diet.

Vegetables that are low in carbs and starch are another great staple of the Keto diet. Veggies are high in nutrients and essential minerals. They're also a great source of fiber, which we all need in our diet. Vegetables also include antioxidants that aid in protection against free radicals that can cause aging.

If you are looking for ways to eat your typical foods while being on the Keto diet, then you will be surprised at what you can do. For instance, cauliflower can be cooked and mimic mashed potatoes, as well as rice. You are even able to make spaghetti noodles out of zucchini.

Cheeses

Cheese is another tasty and nutritious option while on Keto! Who doesn't love a great cheese board and a glass of red wine? Fortunately, all types of cheese are low in carbohydrates and high in fat content. This makes cheese perfect for the Keto diet. For example, just one ounce of cheddar cheese offers only 1 gram of carbohydrates, the protein content is 7 grams, and there is a 20 percent of RDI of calcium.

Cheese is very high in saturated fat; however, it has not been proven to increase heart disease risks. Some studies show that cheese can help against this risk. It also has conjugated linoleic acid. This is a type of fat that is directly linked to weight loss and has also been shown to help the body composition.

Eating cheese regularly will also help the reduction in the loss of your muscle mass, as well as strength when aging is an issue. A 12-week study showed that adults over the age of 50 that ate 7 ounces of ricotta cheese daily had an increase in their muscle mass, as well as muscle strength.

Avocados

Avocados are another great choice! In 3.5 ounces of avocados, about half of an avocado contains 9 grams of carbohydrates. However, 7 of the rams are fiber. This means that the net amount of carbs is 2 grams.

Avocados are incredibly high in many minerals and vitamins. This also includes potassium, a very crucial mineral that many women over the age of 50 are deficient in. A higher level of potassium intake will help make your transition into this diet much easier. Potassium also helps lower the frequency of muscle cramps.

In one study, people who consumed a specially designed diet that included a large number of avocados showed positive changes in their cholesterol. Members experienced a decrease in LDL cholesterol level by 22 percent, as well as triglycerides. They also had an increase in HDL cholesterol by 11 percent.

Poultry and Meat

Poultry and meat are staple foods of almost every diet. Fresh meats and poultry include no carbohydrates and are high in B vitamins. They also contain many different minerals, including zinc, potassium, and selenium.

A study conducted with women over 50 on fatty versus non-fatty meant found that eating a diet in high-fat types of meat increase HDL cholesterol levels by 8% compared to those that ate a low level of fatty meats. It is suggested to only choose to grass-fed meat. That is due to grass-fed animals having more omega-three fats, antioxidants, and linoleum acid.

Eggs are very versatile and are one of the top healthiest foods available. One larger sized egg contains one gram of carbs and less than six grams of protein. This makes eggs an ideal food for someone on the Keto diet.

Eggs are also known to have trigger hormones that will increase the feeling of being full and will keep your blood sugar stable. This will lead to a lower amount of calories consumed in 24 hours. It is essential to consume the whole egg. Most of the nutrients in an egg is found inside of the yolk. It includes zeaxanthin, which aids in the protection of eye health. It also offers a decent amount of antioxidants.

Even though the yolks have a high level of cholesterol, eating eggs does not raise your blood cholesterol levels. This great food shows that it modifies the shape of your LDL and reduces heart disease risks.

Coconut Oil

Coconut oil is unique because it is exceptionally great for those who are on the Keto diet. This product includes medium-chain triglycerides. Unlike long-chain fats, MCTs are absorbed directly by your liver, and then converted into the Ketones or even used as a fast energy resource.

Coconut oil has been utilized to increase the body's Ketone levels in those with Alzheimer's disease, as well as other types of disorders of the nervous system and the brain. The primary fatty type of acid that is in coconut oil is a longer chain fat. It is called lauric acid. It is suggested that the mix of MCTs and lauric acid promotes a constant level of Ketosis. Also, coconut oil promotes the loss of belly fat and aids in weight loss.

Cottage Cheese and Greek Yogurt

Cottage cheese and Greek yogurt are very high in protein. While these items may have some small amounts carbohydrates, they still are included in this diet. For 5 ounces of Greek yogurt offers 5 grams of carbohydrates and 11 grams of protein. The same amount of cottage cheese provides 18 grams of protein, along with 5 grams of carbs.

Both of these products have shown that they help decrease your appetite, and promote a feeling of being full. Cottage cheese and Greek yogurt can be joined with crushed nuts, sugar-free sweetener, or cinnamon.

Olive Oil offers fantastic benefits for your heart. It is very high in oleic acid, as well as monounsaturated fat. This product also provides a lower risk of developing heart disease. In addition, olive oil also offers a high level of antioxidants that are known as phenols. This compound will help further to protect the heart by decreasing any inflammation, as well as improve the artery functions. Olive oil is a pure source of fat, which means it includes no carbs. It is the perfect base for a home-made salad dressing.

Seeds and Nuts

Seeds and nuts are incredibly healthy. They are very low in carbohydrates and high in fat. Frequently eating nuts has been shown to reduce the risk factors of heart disease, depression, cancer, and other chronic type diseases.

Since seeds and nuts are very high in fiber, you will feel fuller, longer. You will absorb fewer calories overall. Even though seeds and nuts are very low in net carbs, the amount will vary drastically depending on the type of seed or nut. For one ounce of a popular nut, it will contain about 28 carbohydrates.

- Almonds: 6 grams of carbs — 3 grams net

- Brazil: 3 grams of carbs — 1 grams net

- Cashews: 9 grams of carbs — 8 grams net

- Macadamia: 4 grams of carbs — 2 grams net

- Pecans: 4 grams of carbs — 1 grams net

- Pistachios: 8 grams of carbs — 5 grams net

- Walnuts: 4 grams of carbs — 2 grams net

- Chia Seeds: 12 grams of carbs — 1 grams net

- Flaxseeds: 8 grams of carbs — 0 grams net

- Pumpkin Seeds: 5 grams of carbs — 4 grams net

- Sesame Seeds: 7 grams of carbs — 3 grams net

Berries

Most of the fruits that are typically eaten are way too high in carbohydrates. Therefore, they are not able to be included in this diet. Berries are the exception. They are very low in carbohydrates and very high in fiber. Blackberries and raspberries have just as much fiber as they do other nutrients.

These two fruits contain a large number of antioxidants and have been known to reduce inflammation and protects against diseases. In a serving size of 3.5 ounces, this list shows you the net content of carbohydrates.

- Blackberries: 10 grams of carbs — 5 grams net

- Blueberries 12 grams of carbs — 12 grams net

- Raspberries: 12 grams of carbs — 6 grams net

- Strawberries: 8 grams of carbs — 6 grams net

Cream and Butter

Cream and butter are great fats to include in your diet. Each of them contains only a few carbs in each serving. For years, cream and butter were believed to contribute or cause heart disease due to their saturated fat content. However, many studies later, it has been proven that many people saturated fat is not linked to heart disease.

Some studies have been conducted that show moderate consumption of dairy may reduce the risk of stroke and heart attacks. Like many other dairy products that are high in fat, cream and butter are very rich in linoleum acid, which promotes fat loss in the body.

Shirataki Noodles

These types of noodles are a great food to eat on the Keto diet. Shirataki noodles are made from viscous fibers called glucomannan. They absorb up to fifty times more weight in water. The viscous fiber will form a gel that will slow down the movement of the food through the digestive tract. This will help decrease the feeling of hunger and reduces sugar spikes. It is a beneficial way to lose weight and manage diabetes. Forms of shirataki noodles include rice, linguine, and fettuccine. They are able to be substituted for other types of noodles in recipes.

Olives

Olives offer the same type of health benefits as olive oil. However, these are in solid form. The main antioxidant in these tasty little Morales is called European. It offers anti-inflammatory properties and can protect the body cells from any damage. In addition, there are studies that show that eating olives will help prevent high blood pressure and bone loss. For one ounce of olives, you will eat 2 grams of carbohydrates, as well as fiber.

Unsweetened Tea and Coffee

Tea and coffee are great healthy drinks that contain no carbs. They do contain caffeine, which increases the body's metabolism and can improve physical performance, mood, and alertness. They have also been shown to reduce diabetes. In fact, it has been proven that people that consume high levels of caffeine have a lower risk of developing diabetes.

Adding in some heavy cream to tea or coffee is acceptable, but you will need to stay away from products that use the word "light." Typically, it is the products that are advertised as non-fat. They contain a lot of carbohydrates.

Cocoa Powder and Dark Chocolate

Cocoa and dark chocolate are delicious and offer a high amount of antioxidants. Cocoa is actually considered a super fruit. Dark chocolate has a large number of flavanols, which reduce heart disease risks. It lowers the blood pressure and will keep your arteries healthy.

Surprisingly, chocolate is able to be included in the Keto diet. However, it is crucial that you eat dark chocolate. It should contain a minimum amount of 70 percent of cocoa solids. One ounce of unsweetened chocolate includes 3 grams of carbohydrates. That means no milk, chocolate candy bars!

Foods to Avoid

All types of sweetened beverages, fruit juices, and other sweetened drinks.

All types of starchy vegetables including white potatoes, sweet potatoes, etc.

Commercial fried foods, snacks, and bakery products including sugar-based desserts.

Wheat pasta, bread, rice, cereals, and other high carb wheat products.

All types of commercial processed food items.

Legumes and beans

Fruits can be consumed but a small quantity

Alcohol and unhealthy cooking oils

Chapter 4: How to choose correct diet plan

If you're concerned about the amount of work and time prep takes, you can save some of the prep for the middle of the week on an evening when you have time.

Be ready to multitask

To speed up the prepping process, get ready to do some multi-tasking. You'll be cooking multiple things at once, and using your oven, stovetop, slow cooker, and any other equipment you have, like a pressure cooker. You can cook multiple things in the oven that have similar temperature and time requirements. Writing out the times, temperatures, and cooking method of what you're making can help you stay organized.

When meal prepping, you should pick your meals 3-5 days in advance, choose simple recipes, prep on a specific day, and learn to multitask.

Have the right containers

A common refrain of meal-prep articles and blogs is that the right containers are essential to productive meal-prepping. If your food isn't stored properly, it can go bad, dry out, get freezer-burn, and so on. Containers are so important that in the next section, we're going to take the time to break down what makes a container the right one.

Resources

Where are you going to find out how to meal prep and what recipes to make? While hopefully this book is your number one resource, it's understandable if you still have a question here or there. We might not be able to guess all the questions you have (though we surely cracked our brains and try our best to!) or can't list everything there is to know about meal prepping in this book. Also, this book doesn't have all the meal prep recipes in the world! So, where do you go from here? Where can you get questions answered and find more recipes? One word, Google!

If you search online for meal prep questions or recipes, you'll be bombarded with hundreds of thousands of options and different websites. It can be overwhelming, which is why this book is so great to have. However, when you're looking for more recipes, there are plentiful online recipes that are delicious and nutritious! Always remember to look at the nutrition facts so that you aren't eating something that may look healthy but actually is not. Pinterest is a website that is a great source for meal prepping. If you aren't familiar with the social networking site, Pinterest now is the time to get acquainted. You can look at lots of different recipes according to your diet. There gluten frees recipes, dairy free recipes, and vegetarian, vegan, and paleo recipes too! If you are looking for specific recipes, definitely look no further than Pinterest. The most exciting feature about Pinterest is that you can save each recipe and organize them into different boards. Think of it as your new online cookbook! There are no limits to the amount of meal prep recipes you will be able to find.

If you would rather have more books in hand, there are tons of cookbooks that focus on meal prepping. This might be slightly more challenging, however, if you have dietary restrictions. We also have a large selection of recipes later on this book that you can pull from. You can make these recipes the start of your meal prep and add in more recipes once you feel you have mastered the ones here.

Food Storage

No one wants his or her food to spoil! Did you know that if your containers are not truly airtight then it could lead to your food going bad much more rapidly? A great recipe is only as good as what it is stored in! Food storage is one of the most important aspects of meal prep. Think of it as another addition to your cooking equipment (which we will talk about a little later in this chapter). If you don't store your food properly, it will spoil quickly and leave your fridge with an unattractive odor that can stink your other food. This is especially important if you are cooking ahead your meals and portioning them out. You will need a lot more containers than normal so be ready to invest in some high-quality containers.

Save yourself more trouble and get a good quality set of food storage items. Food storage containers that are cheap typically comes with low-quality sealing materials that do not last very long and leave you spending more money in the long run as you have to replace them.

Plastic Food Sealing Bags

The first item for food storage you will need is plastic food sealing bags. Plastic food sealing bags are about to become your best friend! Plastic sealing bags of all different sizes are great to portion out your snacks or take some breakfast on the go. Ziploc food bags are good options. For your snack and breakfast, try to get sandwich sized sealing bags. This will help you to be able to quickly grab your snacks as you head out the door. The best part about sandwich sized bags is you can squeeze out the air and make them air tight to ensure your food stays fresh! You won't need these plastic bags for meals; these are only going to be used for snacks or breakfast items like muffins.

Plastic Freezer Bags

In addition to sandwich sized plastic sealing bags, you'll also need gallon sized freezer bags. When you prep your freezer meals, gallon size bags are an absolute must. They are super easy to write on with a permanent marker so that you won't forget how to cook it and how long to cook it. You can also write the name of the recipe on the gallon size bag so you can easily find the recipe you are searching for. Don't forget to write down the date you froze the recipe so you know to consume it within a 4-month period before turning bad. As a great tip to share on storing your freezer meals, you can squeeze out the air and lay them flat in your freezer so that they occupy minimal space. Then you can stack freezer meals on top of each other in order of "First in First Out" rule to keep your fridge organized and have your frozen food ingredients easily accessible.

Plastic and Glass Food Containers

For the days that you cook everything for the week in advance, solid storage containers are not to be missed. The last thing you need is for all your prepped meals to go bad because your containers were not up to requirements. There are two different types of containers to get. You can have glass or plastic storage containers. Stay away from stainless steel containers. While they make great storage containers, you cannot microwave them and so they don't have much of a place in a meal prep household.

Make sure to get a few different sized containers so that you portion each meal correctly and don't run out of room. Whether you choose to use glass containers or plastic containers, it's a personal preference. While plastic may cheaper than glass, some people are afraid that the chemicals in plastic can leach into your food while you reheat it. Plastic containers can also warp easily in the dishwasher. If your containers have warped, they need to be thrown out because they are no longer airtight. Glass doesn't stain, is easy to clean, and doesn't keep odors like plastic might. But while glass containers ensure that the chemicals from plastic don't leach into your food, they can be a little heavy to carry around. Glass will last longer than plastic if you do not drop them. Weigh the pros and cons between the two different types of containers and choose the option that best works for your lifestyle.

Food Vacuum Sealer Bags

If you want to buy in bulk and keep your meats as fresh as possible, vacuum sealed bags can help with this. Vacuum sealer bags take out all the air from the bag so your food stays fresh longer. Keeping food fresh isn't their only benefit. When you vacuum seal your food, it saves you space. It makes the bag go so tightly around your prepped meal or meat that you do not need to worry about freezer space. This is a great addition if you are doing the freezer style meal prep. You can use vacuum bags of the similar required size for your portioning and this helps so much in organizing your freezer as well.

There are plenty of brands for Food Vacuum Sealing system selling in the market. Food Saver is one of the more popular and reliable brands that you may consider. It offers very decent sealing result and the food stored can last 2 to 3 times longer as compared to non-vacuum sealing methods in the freezer.

Cooking Wares

If you are cooking frequently, chances are you have an arsenal of cooking equipment that you already use at your disposal. However, if you are just starting out your cooking affairs, you may have little to nothing for your kitchen. This is especially true for new college students or newly-wed couples. With meal prepping, you will need a few different equipment to cook with. The good news is meal prepping doesn't require anything special in the kitchen. Everything you will buy can be used over and over or all you're cooking needs! It's time to go shopping!

Measuring Cups and Spoons

The most basic item required is a set of measuring cups and measuring spoons. You are going to be cooking a lot of different recipes and a good recipe depends on measurements. If you try to guess the measurements in a recipe you'll end up with a less than desired meal. These measuring cups do not need to be anything fancy, grab the cheapest pair you can find and those will work! Make sure to have a set of cups that go from 1/4 cup to 1 cup, and a set of spoons that go from ¼ teaspoon to 1 tablespoon. You can find measuring cups and spoons at any grocery store and even at the dollar store.

Besides the measuring cups and spoons, you'll also need a few cooking utensils. Your cooking utensils will make your cooking go much easier and enjoyable. You don't want to be caught without a few good spatulas. Look for a spatula that you can use to scrape the sides of bowls for sauces and mixes. You'll also need a spatula that you can turn and lift with (the kind you need for pancakes!). In addition to these two spatulas, make sure you have other basic utensils like a whisk, a ladle, and a serving spoon.

Cooking Pots and Pans

You can't cook without items for the stove and oven! Let's talk about pots and pans. A good set of pots and pans is surely a great asset for an aspiring meal prepper. You'll be cooking a lot! Our favorite pan is a trusty cast iron skillet. Cast iron skillets are cheap but they last forever. They hold their heat amazingly well and are great non-stick pans once they are seasoned correctly. They also create the perfect sear and greatly mimic a grill if you want grilled chicken or a hearty steak. They can also be placed in the oven to help you roast veggies and meats as well. And the best part about them is that they aren't too expensive! You can get a great cast iron skillet for around $25. Make sure you have at least two skillets and two pots. The pots will be used for cooking your grains and for steaming your veggies. They can also be used to make your sauces. You can use any pots you already may have but we recommend having a smaller saucepan and a pot large enough to cook your grains.

Knives and Cutting Equipment

If you plan on eating healthy, there's one kitchen tool you absolutely must have: a knife set. Meal prepping really cannot be done without a good knife set. You are going to be chopping up a ton of fruits and vegetables so make sure you have a trusty knife set and a few different cutting boards. There are a lot of different types of knives and multiple materials knives are made from. Stainless steel knives are sharp, easy to use, and heavy duty. If you have a set of stainless steel knives, there's no reason to replace them! If you haven't purchased a knife set yet, be aware that stainless steel can rust. Ceramic knives are a lot lighter than your traditional steel and they are super sharp. Just make sure you know what you are doing before you start chopping with ceramic. Ceramic knives can shatter if dropped or cut through something too hard. They are fairly cheap and they do not rust so they make a great choice if you want to try something new. If you don't want to buy a whole knife set, make sure you have at least the basic knives. Make sure to have a chef knife, a knife with a serrated edge, and a boning knife. We also recommend that you have a vegetable peeler. You may need to peel vegetables like potatoes, sweet potatoes, and squashes so we recommend you do not skip purchasing a vegetable peeler. You don't have to spend hundreds of dollars on new knives; you can get a new set of knives for around $50 that will certainly last you a while.

Oven Wares

You didn't think you could meal prep without roasting items, did you? Here comes that trusty cookie sheet! A cookie sheet is an absolute must with meal prepping. We use cookie sheets to roast our veggies then cookour protein on days we aren't using our pots/pans/slow cookers. An average size cookie sheet (size 13"x18") will be large enough to successfully cook whatever you need to. You can get a silicone baking mat to accompany your cookie sheet or just use parchment paper. This will help you save time on clean up and you won't have to scrub the cookie sheet after every single use. The baking mat and parchment paper is optional but you will appreciate it after trying cooking without it.

Cooking Equipment

With all the wonderful recipes researched and ingredients nicely prepared, you're going to have it cooked. Different recipes call for different cooking methods thus the cooking apparatus vary. Following section brings to you the various cooking apparatus and explains how they can be used efficiently in your meal prep journey.

Stove Top & Induction Cooktop

To sauté, boil, fry, or steam, you will need a stove top. Your stove can either be gas, electric, or induction. Most homes will come equipped with a few different sized stove tops. However, if you do not have a home that comes with a stove top, you can buy a portable induction cooktop. These can be as small as a single stove top and you can purchase one for around $50. You won't be able to meal prep without it.

Slow Cooker

If you are planning on doing any freezer meal prep, your most important tool is going to be your slow cooker. If you don't have a slow cooker, go out and buy one, it's about to become your new best friend! Slow cookers are extremely versatile and you can buy a new one for as little as $15. Slow cookers will make your meals taste like a million dollars without you lifting a finger. Even if you aren't planning on doing any freezer meals, a slow cooker can help you out with your prep work. You can put protein in the slow cooker in the morning and a few hours later you have tender and amazing meat for the rest of the week. This is one piece of equipment you won't regret buying.

Convection Oven

Convection ovens are great little tools. They can be set up on your counter but will be able to bake or roast whatever you need for meal prepping. The best part about convection ovens are that they are evenly heated. You won't have some parts of your meal burnt while the other is still raw!

Microwave

To reheat your meals, a microwave is a must. This is what makes meal prepping so great! Once you have prepped your meals, you stick it in the microwave for just a few minutes. Microwaves can be installed in your home or you can get a counter one for as little as $30.

Pressure Cooker

Today pressure cookers are becoming even more popular. They have been around for some time but nowadays there are electric pressure cookers which make cooking so much faster and convenient. Whether you have a traditional stove top pressure cooker or an electric, it can make recipes a lot easier. It can cut down your cooking time by hours. Think shredded chicken in as little as 15 minutes! If you forget to put your meal in the slow cooker, your pressure cooker can usually take that frozen meal then cook it in under an hour. It also makes rice, beans, and other grains very quickly. This is highly recommended cooking equipment in your kitchen if you value time more than anything else. Instant Pot and Power Pressure Cooker XL are two popular choices in the market now.

Electric Lunch Box

If you want to keep your meals warm, an electric lunch box can help. Maybe you don't have a microwave at work or you just want it ready immediately at lunch time! An electric lunch box can plug into your desk and warm up your food so it is ready by the time noon rolls around. Whether you are at an office or on the road, there are many different electric lunch boxes to choose from. Some plug into a standard wall plug but they also have ones that can plug into your car or plug into the USB port on your computer or laptop. Some electric lunch box models also come with cooking function which means you can have your rice, porridge or even stews and soup cooked. Advanced features like auto timer for cooking start/stop timing are also available for higher end models.

Chapter 5: 30 days Meal Plan

Day 1

Breakfast- Buttered Basil on Scrambled Egg

Lunch- Hashed Brussels Sprouts

Dinner- Cheese Mushroom Spinach Quiche

Day 2

Breakfast- Mushroom Omelet Keto Approved

Lunch- Stir-Fried Ground Beef

Dinner- Zucchini Carrot Patties

Day 3

Breakfast- Caprese Omelet Keto Approved

Lunch- Keto Carrot Cake

Dinner- Tomato Zucchini Frittata

Day 4

Breakfast- Keto Approved Pancakes

Lunch- Asparagus Gremolata

Dinner- Italian Basil Tomato Omelet

Day 5

Breakfast- Keto Approved Easy Egg Muffins

Lunch- Beets with Yogurt

Dinner- Curried Spinach

Day 6

Breakfast- Keto Asparagus Frittata

Lunch- Vegetarian Faux Stew

Dinner- Tofu Scramble

Day 7

Breakfast- Keto-Approved Blueberry Pancakes

Lunch- Egg Fried Cauli Rice

Dinner- Cheese Herb Frittata

Day 8

Breakfast- Slow Cooked Egg Casserole

Lunch- Vegetable en Papillote

Dinner- Easy Broccoli Omelet

Day 9

Breakfast- Breakfast Cauliflower Hash

Lunch- Keto Coconut Almond Cake

Dinner- Leek Mushroom Frittata

Day 10

Breakfast- Keto Approved Coco-Porridge

Lunch- Faux Beet Risotto

Dinner- Broccoli Cream Cheese Quiche

Day 11

Breakfast- Buttered Basil on Scrambled Egg

Lunch- Hashed Brussels Sprouts

Dinner- Cheese Mushroom Spinach Quiche

Day 12

Breakfast- Mushroom Omelet Keto Approved

Lunch- Stir-Fried Ground Beef

Dinner- <u>Zucchini Carrot Patties</u>

Day 13

Breakfast- <u>Caprese Omelet Keto Approved</u>

Lunch- <u>Keto Carrot Cake</u>

Dinner- <u>Tomato Zucchini Frittata</u>

Day 14

Breakfast- <u>Keto Approved Pancakes</u>

Lunch- <u>Asparagus Gremolata</u>

Dinner- <u>Italian Basil Tomato Omelet</u>

Day 15

Breakfast- <u>Keto Approved Easy Egg Muffins</u>

Lunch- <u>Beets with Yogurt</u>

Dinner- <u>Curried Spinach</u>

Day 16

Breakfast- <u>Keto Asparagus Frittata</u>

Lunch- <u>Vegetarian Faux Stew</u>

Dinner- Tofu Scramble

Day 17

Breakfast- Keto-Approved Blueberry Pancakes

Lunch- Egg Fried Cauli Rice

Dinner- Cheese Herb Frittata

Day 18

Breakfast- Slow Cooked Egg Casserole

Lunch- Vegetable en Papillote

Dinner- Easy Broccoli Omelet

Day 19

Breakfast- Breakfast Cauliflower Hash

Lunch- Keto Coconut Almond Cake

Dinner- Leek Mushroom Frittata

Day 20

Breakfast- Keto Approved Coco-Porridge

Lunch- Faux Beet Risotto

Dinner- Broccoli Cream Cheese Quiche

Day 21

Breakfast- Buttered Basil on Scrambled Egg

Lunch- Hashed Brussels Sprouts

Dinner- Cheese Mushroom Spinach Quiche

Day 22

Breakfast- Mushroom Omelet Keto Approved

Lunch- Stir-Fried Ground Beef

Dinner- Zucchini Carrot Patties

Day 23

Breakfast- Caprese Omelet Keto Approved

Lunch- Keto Carrot Cake

Dinner- Tomato Zucchini Frittata

Day 24

Breakfast- Keto Approved Pancakes

Lunch- Asparagus Gremolata

Dinner- Italian Basil Tomato Omelet

Day 25

Breakfast- Keto Approved Easy Egg Muffins

Lunch- Beets with Yogurt

Dinner- Curried Spinach

Day 26

Breakfast- Keto Asparagus Frittata

Lunch- Vegetarian Faux Stew

Dinner- Tofu Scramble

Day 27

Breakfast- Keto-Approved Blueberry Pancakes

Lunch- Egg Fried Cauli Rice

Dinner- Cheese Herb Frittata

Day 28

Breakfast- Slow Cooked Egg Casserole

Lunch- Vegetable en Papillote

Dinner- Easy Broccoli Omelet

Day 29

Breakfast- Breakfast Cauliflower Hash

Lunch- Keto Coconut Almond Cake

Dinner- Leek Mushroom Frittata

Day 30

Breakfast- Keto Approved Coco-Porridge

Lunch- Faux Beet Risotto

Dinner- Broccoli Cream Cheese Quiche

Chapter 6: Shopping list

The last step to adopting a keto diet is for you to make a shopping list and go out to shop for keto friendly foods.

So how can you execute this step?

The first thing that you will need to do when executing this step is to get rid of every keto unfriendly food in your house and in your office.

So take a big bag, go to your kitchen and slowly start placing every food that is not allowed on a keto diet on that bag. Go to your office and repeat the exercise.

At the end of the whole exercise, you can either throw all the foods away or you can donate them to family, friends or those that are in need of food.

Now that your kitchen is free from keto unfriendly foods, it's time for you to sit down and come up with a shopping list that will restock your kitchen with keto friendly foods.

As you write your shopping list, consult the keto friendly food list that you learnt in the previous step.

Once done, hit the market and use the shopping list to shop. Restock your kitchen and start cooking keto friendly meals that will change your health and wellbeing.

Sage Leaves

Cloves Garlic

Onion

Olive Oil

Red Potatoes

Black Beans

Parsley

Swiss Chard

Sea Salt & Black Pepper

Water

Flaxseeds

Coconut Oil

Vanilla Vegan Powder

Baking Powder

Carrot

Avocado

Poppy seeds

Lemon juice

Ginger

Strawberries

Stevia

Coconut flakes

Paprika

Blueberries

Banana

Almond milk

Chia seeds

Lentils

Tomatoes

Okra

Broccoli

Egg

Chicken

Bacon

Beef

Rice

Shrimp

Chapter 7: Breakfast Recipes

Buttered Basil on Scrambled Egg

Total time: 13 minutes

Ingredients

- 2 oz. butter

- 4 eggs

- 4 tbsp coconut cream or coconut milk or sour cream

- 4 tbsp fresh basil

- salt

Directions:

Place a nonstick pan on low heat and melt butter.

Meanwhile, in a small bowl whisk eggs, coconut cream, basil and salt. Pour in pan.

With a spatula, stir eggs until scrambled and cooked to desired doneness.

Let it cool. Evenly divide into suggested servings and place in meal prep containers.

Mushroom Omelet Keto Approved

Total time: 18 minutes

Ingredients:

- 9 eggs

- 2/3 yellow onion

- 3 oz. butter, for frying

- 3 oz. shredded cheese

- 9 mushrooms

- salt and pepper

Directions:

Place a nonstick skillet on medium heat.

Meanwhile, in a large bowl whisk well eggs, salt, and pepper.

Add butter to pan and let it melt.

Add mushrooms and onion. Sauté for 3 minutes. Pour in eggs.

Cover and lower heat to medium low. Cook for 8 minutes.

Add cheese on top. Cover and continue to cook for another 3 minutes.

Fold in half and continue cooking until eggs are golden brown underneath.

Let it cool. Evenly divide into suggested servings and place in meal prep containers.

Caprese Omelet Keto Approved

 Total time: 25 minutes

Ingredients:

- 9 eggs

- 1½ tbsp fresh basil or dried basil

- 3 tbsp olive oil

- 4½ oz. cherry tomatoes cut in halves or tomatoes cut in halves

- 7½ oz. fresh mozzarella cheese

- salt and pepper

Directions:

Place a large nonstick pan on medium heat and heat oil.

Meanwhile, in a large bowl whisk eggs. Season with salt and pepper. Mix well.

Add sliced tomatoes in pan and sauté for 4 minutes.

Pour eggs in pan. Lower heat to medium low, cover and cook for 5 minutes.

Add cheese and continue cooking while covered until omelet is set, around 8 minutes more.

Let it cool. Evenly divide into suggested servings and place in meal prep containers.

Keto Approved Pancakes

Total time: 15 minutes

Ingredients:

- 8 eggs

- 2¾ oz. pork rinds

- 4 tsp ground cinnamon

- 4 tsp maple extract

- 8 tbsp coconut oil, for frying

- 8 tbsp unsweetened cashew milk

- 2 tbsp coconut oil

Directions:

In a blender, pulse pork rids until it becomes a fine powder. Add remaining ingredients and blend well to combine.

Place a small nonstick skillet on medium heat and heat a tablespoon of coconut oil.

Once hot add ¼ cup of batter and cook for two minutes. Flip pancake and cook the other side for another minute.

Repeat process until you have used up all the batter.

Let it cool. Evenly divide into suggested servings and place in meal prep containers.

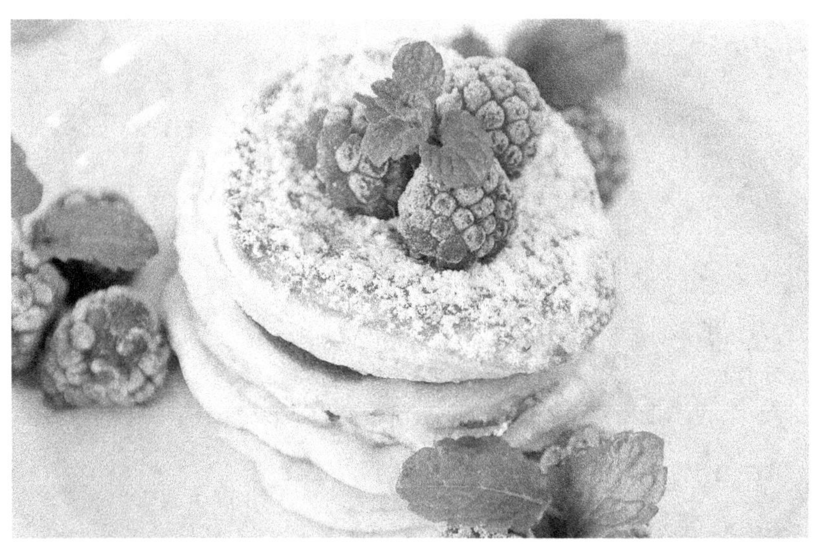

Keto Approved Easy Egg Muffins

Total time: 25 minutes

Ingredients:

- 12 eggs

- 2 scallions, finely chopped

- 2 tbsp red pesto or green pesto (optional)

- 5 oz. air-dried chorizo or cooked bacon, chopped or crumbled

- 6 oz. shredded cheese

- salt and pepper

Directions:

Lightly grease 12 muffin tins and preheat oven to 350ºF.

Evenly sprinkle scallions and chorizo or bacon on bottom of tins.

In a bowl, whisk eggs. Season with pepper and salt. Add pesto and cheese. Mix well.

Evenly pour eggs in muffin tins.

Pop in the oven and bake for 18 minutes or until set.

Let it cool. Evenly divide into suggested servings and place in meal prep containers.

Keto Asparagus Frittata

Total time: 28 minutes

Ingredients:

- 8 Eggs

- Salt and Freshly Ground Black Pepper to Taste

- 1/2 Cup Grated Parmesan Cheese

- 1 Tablespoon Olive Oil

- 2 Teaspoons Butter

- 1/2-Pound Asparagus, Trimmed,

- 7 Tablespoons Milk

Directions:

Place a nonstick pan on medium heat and add oil.

Once oil is hot, sauté asparagus for 10 minutes or until tender.

Meanwhile, in a bowl whisk eggs until frothy. Season with pepper and salt. Stir in milk and cheese.

Pour egg mixture into pan with asparagus, lower heat to medium low, cover pan, and cook for 12 minutes or until eggs are set.

Let it cool. Evenly divide into suggested servings and place in meal prep containers.

Keto-Approved Blueberry Pancakes

Total time: 10 minutes

Ingredients:

- 1 egg

- 1 pinch salt

- 1 tbsp almond milk

- 1 tbsp coconut oil

- 1 tsp coconut flour

- 1/16 tsp Stevia

- 1/4 cup almond flour

- 1/4 tsp baking powder

- 1/4 tsp cinnamon

- ¼ cup blueberries

Directions:

In blender, mix all ingredients except for blueberries and coconut oil. Blend until smooth and creamy.

In a small nonstick pan on medium heat, heat ½ of the oil.

Once oil is hot, add half of the batter. Drop half of the blueberries in a single layer in the cooking pancake. Cook for 1 ½ minutes. Flip pancake and cook for another minute.

Repeat process to remaining batter.

Let it cool. Evenly divide into suggested servings and place in meal prep containers.

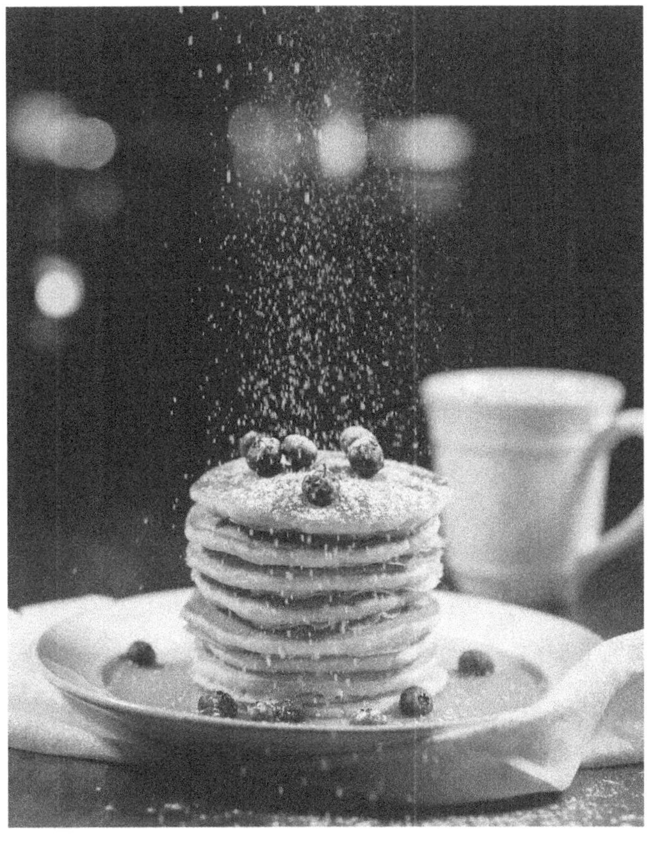

Slow Cooked Egg Casserole

Total time: 5 hours 10 minutes

Ingredients:

- 12 eggs, whisked

- ½ cup feta cheese

- ½ cup milk

- ½ cup sun dried tomatoes

- ½ teaspoon salt

- 1 cup baby Bella mushrooms (sliced)

- 1 tablespoon red onion, chopped

- 1 teaspoon black pepper

- 1 teaspoon garlic, minced

- 2 cups spinach

Directions:

In a large bowl, whisk eggs.

Season with pepper and salt.

Mix in milk, garlic, and red onion.

Mix thoroughly in spinach, mushrooms, and sun-dried tomatoes.

With cooking spray, grease sides and bottom of a slow cooker.

Cover and cook on low for 5 hours or until eggs are set.

Let it cool. Evenly divide into suggested servings and place in meal prep containers.

Breakfast Cauliflower Hash

Total time: 25 minutes

Ingredients:

- 8-ounce shaved red pastrami, chopped into 1-inch slices

- ½ green bell pepper, chopped into ¼-inch pieces

- 1 teaspoon Cajun seasoning

- 1-pound bag frozen cauliflower, chopped roughly

- 2 tablespoons minced garlic

- ½ onion, chopped into ¼-inch pieces

- 2 tablespoons olive oil

Directions:

In a blender or food processor, add roughly chopped cauliflower and burr until you have even rice-like flakes. Set aside.

Place a medium nonstick pan on medium heat and add oil.

Once oil is hot, stir in garlic and cook until lightly browned, around 2 minutes.

Stir in onions and Cajun seasoning. Sauté for a minute.

Add burred cauliflower and sauté for 5 minutes or until lightly browned.

Stir in green pepper and pastrami.

Continue sautéing for another 5 minutes and then turn off heat.

Let it cool. Evenly divide into suggested servings and place in meal prep containers.

Keto Approved Coco-Porridge

Total time: 15 minutes

Ingredients:

- 2 eggs

- 1 tsp ground psyllium husk

- 2 tablespoons coconut flour

- 2-ounces butter

- 8 tablespoons coconut cream

- Salt to taste

Directions:

Place a medium pot on medium heat.

Melt butter. Once melted add all ingredients and mix well.

Bring to a simmer while stirring pot every now and then.

Once simmering, continuously mix pot until desired thickness is achieved.

Turn off heat.

Let it cool. Evenly divide into suggested servings and place in meal prep containers.

Mexican Egg Casserole

Total time: 25 minutes

Ingredients:

- 10 eggs

- ¼ teaspoon pepper

- ¼ teaspoon salt

- ½ teaspoon coriander

- ½ teaspoon garlic powder

- 1 cup milk

- 1 cup pepper jack

- 1 cup salsa

- 1 teaspoon chili powder

- 1 teaspoon cumin

- 12-ounces Jones Dairy Farm Pork Sausage Roll

Directions:

Place a heavy-bottomed pot on medium heat.

Once pot is hot, add pork sausage and cook until no longer pink.

Stir in chili powder, cumin, coriander, and garlic powder and sauté for a minute.

Pour in salsa, mix well, and press warming button.

Meanwhile, in a large bowl whisk well eggs, milk, pepper, and salt.

Pour egg mixture into Instant Pot and mix well.

Add cheese, whisk well.

Cover and cook for 8 minutes on medium heat.

Lower heat to medium low and continue cooking until casserole has set, around 12 to 15 minutes. Do not open lid.

Let it cool. Evenly divide into suggested servings and place in meal prep containers.

Mushroom-Kale Frittata

Total time: 27 minutes

Ingredients:

- 4 large eggs, beaten

- 2 tablespoons ghee

- 2 teaspoons minced garlic

- 1 cup mushrooms, sliced

- 1 cup chopped kale

- Pepper and salt to taste

Directions:

Place a medium skillet on medium heat and heat oil.

Meanwhile, in a bowl whisk well the eggs. Season with pepper and salt to taste.

Sauté garlic for a minute.

Add mushrooms and sauté for 5 minutes.

Add kale and sauté for 2 minutes or until nearly wilted.

Pour in eggs, cover, and cook for 5 minutes.

Lower heat to medium low and cook for another 5 minutes or until set.

Let it cool. Evenly divide into suggested servings and place in meal prep containers.

Keto Spinach Frittata

Total time: 27 minutes

Ingredients:

- 8 large eggs, beaten

- ¼ onion, diced

- 1 cup almond milk, unsweetened

- 2 cups spinach

- 4 large egg whites, beaten

- 1 tbsp oil

Directions:

Place a medium cast-iron pan on medium high heat and heat oil.

In a mixing bowl, combine the eggs, egg whites, and almond milk. Season with salt and pepper to taste.

Add onions to pan and sauté for 3 minutes.

Stir in spinach and sauté for a minute. Then, evenly spread all over the pan.

Pour in egg mixture.

Cover and cook for 8 minutes.

Lower heat to medium low and continue cooking for another 10 minutes or until Frittata is set.

Let it cool. Evenly divide into suggested servings and place in meal prep containers.

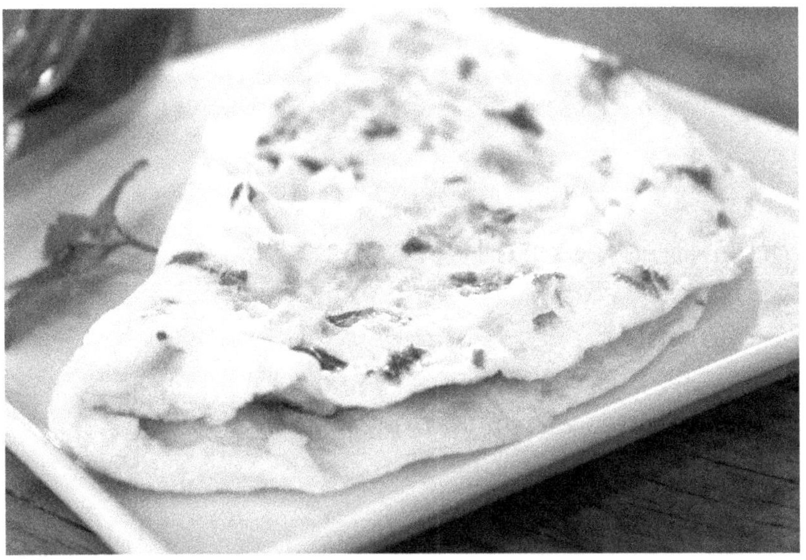

Breakfast Taco on a Skillet

Total time: 55 minutes

Ingredients:

- 10 large eggs

- 1/4 cup sour cream

- 1 1/2 cups shredded sharp cheddar cheese, divided

- 1 roma tomato, diced

- 2 tablespoons torn fresh cilantro (optional)

- 1/4 cup heavy cream

- 1/4 cup salsa

- 1-pound ground beef

- 2 green onions, sliced

- 2/3 cup water

- 4 tablespoons Taco Seasoning

- 1/4 cup sliced black olives

Directions:

Place a large cast-iron pan on medium-high heat.

Once hot, add beef and sauté until browned, around 10 minutes. Drain excess oil.

Add water and taco seasoning to pan and mix well. Lower heat to medium and continue cooking until water has evaporated, around 10 minutes more.

Preheat oven to 375ºF.

Meanwhile, in a bowl whisk the eggs. Stir in heavy cream and a cup of cheese. Mix well.

Transfer half of the meat on a plate.

Pour egg in pan and mix well.

Pop the pan in the oven and bake until cooked through, around 30 minutes.

Remove from oven and top with salsa, sour cream, green onion, cilantro, olives, tomato, and the remaining cheese.

Let it cool. Evenly divide into suggested servings and place in meal prep containers.

Keto Approved Homemade Hot Pockets

Total time: 40 minutes

Ingredients:

- 4 eggs large

- 4 tablespoon unsalted butter

- 6 slices bacon cooked

- 1 1/2 cup Mozzarella

- 2/3 cup almond flour

Directions:

Place a nonstick skillet and place on medium heat. Cook bacon for 5 minutes, divide into 4 equal parts and set aside.

Whisk eggs in a bowl, season with salt and pepper. Cook in same pan. Transfer to a plate and divide evenly into four.

Preheat oven to 400°F.

In a microwave safe bowl, melt mozzarella and butter. Stir in flour and mix well.

Roll dough in two sheets of wax paper into ¼-inch thickness. Divide into 4 equal sizes.

Place ¼ egg and ¼ bacon in middle of one dough. Fold in half and seal edges. Poke the middle in several spots to vent hot pockets. Repeat process for remaining dough.

Place on a lightly greased baking sheet and bake in the oven until golden brown, around 20 minutes.

Let it cool. Evenly divide into suggested servings and place in meal prep containers.

Egg Cups Wrapped in Zucchini

Total time: 45 minutes

Ingredients:

- 8 eggs

- 1 cup Pinch red pepper flakes

- 1 cup shredded cheddar

- 1/2 cup cherry tomatoes, quartered

- 1/2 cup heavy cream

- 1/2 tsp dried oregano

- ¼-lb ham, chopped

- 2 zucchini, peeled into strips

- Cooking spray, for pan

- Freshly ground black pepper

- Kosher salt

Directions:

With cooking spray, lightly grease 12 muffin tins. Preheat oven to 400°F.

To form cups, line the muffin tins with the zucchini strips. Ensuring that it forms like a muffin cup.

Sprinkle cherry tomatoes and ham in the cups.

Whisk well heavy cream, eggs, red pepper flakes, and oregano in a medium bowl. Season with pepper and salt. Mix well.

Evenly divide egg mixture into the 12 muffin tins.

Pop in the oven and bake for 30 minutes or until eggs are set.

Let it cool. Evenly divide into suggested servings and place in meal prep containers.

Traditional Scotch Eggs Recipe

Total time: 20 minutes

Ingredients:

- ½ teaspoon paprika powder

- 1 ½ pounds ground pork

- 1 egg, beaten

- 1 garlic clove minced

- 5 eggs, hardboiled and peeled

Directions:

Place a steam rack in the Instant Pot and pour a cup of water.

Combine the beaten egg, ground pork, garlic, and paprika in a mixing bowl. Season with salt and pepper to taste.

Divide the meat mixture into 5 balls.

Flatten the balls with your hands and place an egg at the center. Cover the egg with the meat mixture. Do the same thing with the other balls.

Allow to set in the fridge for at least 2 hours.

Place the frozen meat on the steam rack.

Close the lid and make sure that the vent points to "Sealing."

Press the "Steam" button and adjust the time to 15 minutes.

Do natural pressure release and allow the balls to cool in the fridge for an hour.

Take the steam rack out and thrown away the water.

Without the lid on, press the Sauté button and allow the balls to sear on all sides until lightly golden.

Let it cool. Evenly divide into suggested servings and place in meal prep containers.

Chapter 8: Lunch Recipes

Hashed Brussels Sprouts

Total time: 45 minutes

Ingredients:

- 1/4 tsp red pepper flakes

- 4 large eggs

- Freshly ground black pepper

- 6 slices bacon, cut into 1" pieces

- kosher salt

- 2 tbsp water

- 2 garlic cloves, minced

- 1/2 onion, chopped

- 1-lb Brussels sprouts, trimmed and quartered

Directions:

On medium heat, place a nonstick pan and crisp fry bacon. Once done, transfer to a plate and pat away the oil with a paper towel.

In same pan with bacon grease, sauté onion for a minute.

Stir in Brussels sprouts and cook for 3 minutes.

Season with red pepper flakes, pepper, and salt.

Add water and continue cooking until liquid has evaporated.

Create four holes in the pan and crack eggs. Season eggs with pepper and salt.

Cover and continue cooking until eggs are cooked to desired doneness.

Let it cool. Evenly divide into suggested servings and place in meal prep containers.

Stir-Fried Ground Beef

Total time: 20 minutes

Ingredients:

- 1-lb ground beef

- ½ cup broccoli, chopped

- ½ of medium-sized onions, chopped

- ½ of medium-sized red bell pepper, chopped

- 1 tbsp cayenne pepper (optional)

- 1 tbsp Chinese five spices

- 1 tbsp coconut oil

- 2 kale leaves, chopped

- 5 medium-sized mushrooms, sliced

Directions:

In a skillet, heat the coconut oil over medium high heat.

Sauté the onions for one minute and add the vegetables while stirring constantly.

Add the ground beef and the spices.

Cook for two minutes and reduce the heat to medium.

Cover the skillet and continue to cook the beef and vegetables for another 10 minutes.

Let it cool. Evenly divide into suggested servings and place in meal prep containers.

Keto Carrot Cake

Total time: 75 minutes

Ingredients

5 Eggs

1 ¼ cup Almond flour

½ cup Swerve Sweetener

1 tsp Baking Powder

1 ½ tsp Apple Pie Spice

⅓ cup Coconut Oil

½ cup Heavy Cream

1 ½ cup Carrots, shredded

⅓ cup Walnuts, chopped

2 cups Water

Directions

Grease an 8-inch cake tin; set aside. Place all ingredients in a bowl, and mix evenly with a cake mixer. Pour the batter into the cake tin and cover the tin with foil. A pinch the edges of the pan to tighten the foil. Pour the water into the Instant Pot and fit in a trivet with handles.

Place the tin on top. Seal the lid, select Cake mode for 40 minutes on High. Once ready, do a natural release for 10 minutes; then quickly release the pressure. Let cool before slicing.

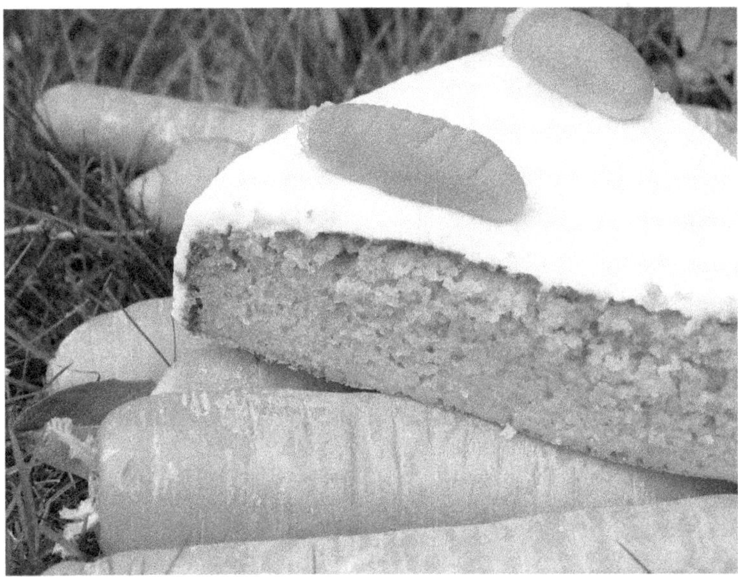

Asparagus Gremolata

Total time: 30 minutes

Ingredients:

1 lb Asparagus, hard ends cut off

1 cup Water

Gremolata:

2 Lemons, zested

2 Oranges, zested

4 cloves Garlic, minced

½ cup Chopped Parsley

Salt to taste

Pepper to taste

Directions

Mix all gremolata ingredients in a bowl; set aside. Pour water in the pot and fit a steamer basket. Add asparagus to the basket, seal the lid and cook on Steam for 4 minutes on High.

Once ready, quickly release the pressure. Remove asparagus and serve with gremolata.

Beets with Yogurt

Total time: 55 minutes

Ingredients:

1 lb Beets, washed

1 Lime, zested and juiced

1 cup Plain Full Milk Yogurt

1 clove Garlic, minced

Salt to taste

1 tbsp Fresh Dill, chopped

1 tbsp Olive oil to drizzle

Black Pepper to garnish

1 cup Water

Directions

Pour the water in the Instant Pot and fit in a steamer basket. Add the beets, seal the lid, secure the pressure valve and select Manual mode on High Pressure mode for 30 minutes.

Once ready, do a natural pressure release for 10 minutes, then quickly release the remaining pressure. Remove the beets to a bowl to cool, and then remove the skin. Cut into wedges.

Place beets in a dip plate, drizzle the olive oil and lime juice over; set aside. In a bowl, mix garlic, yogurt and lime zest. Pour over the beets and garnish with black pepper, salt, and dill.

Vegetarian Faux Stew

Total time: 35 minutes

Ingredients:

1 ½ cups Diced Tomatoes

4 cloves Garlic

1 tsp Minced Ginger

1 tsp Turmeric

1 tsp Cayenne Powder

2 tsp Paprika

Salt to taste

1 tsp Cumin Powder

2 cups Dry Soy Curls

1 ½ cups Water

3 tbsp Butter

½ cup Heavy Cream

¼ cup Chopped Cilantro

Directions

Place the tomatoes, water, soy curls and all spices in the Instant Pot. Seal the lid, secure the pressure valve and select Manual mode on High Pressure mode for 6 minutes.

Once ready, do a natural pressure release for 10 minutes. Select Sauté, add the cream and butter. Stir while crushing the tomatoes with the back of the spoon. Stir in the cilantro and serve.

Egg Fried Cauli Rice

Total time: 25 minutes

Ingredients:

2 heads Cauliflower, cut in big chunks

8 Eggs, beaten

3 tbsp Butter

5 cloves Garlic, minced

1 large White Onion, chopped

2 tsp Olive oil

2 tsp Soy Sauce

Salt to taste

½ cup Water

Directions

Pour water in the Instant Pot and fit in a steamer basket. Place the cauli chunks in the basket. Seal the lid and cook on High Pressure for 1 minute. Once ready, quickly release the pressure.

Remove the cauli chunks onto a plate. Discard the water in the pot and clean dry. Select Sauté, and melt olive oil and butter. Add the eggs and stir frequently to break as they cook.

Add onions and garlic, stir and cook for 2 minutes. Add cauli chunks, and use a masher to break the chunks into a rice-like consistency. Stir in soy sauce and salt, and cook for 3 more minutes. Serve cauli rice as a side dish.

Vegetable en Papillote

Total time: 25 minutes

Ingredients:

1 cup Green Beans

4 small Carrots, widely julienned

¼ tsp Black Pepper

A pinches Salt

1 clove Garlic, crushed

2 tbsp Butter

2 slices Lemon

1 tbsp Chopped Thyme

1 tbsp Oregano

1 tbsp Chopped Parsley

17 inch Parchment Paper

Directions

Add all ingredients, except lemon slices and butter, in a bowl and toss. Place the paper on a flat surface and add the mixed ingredients at the center of the paper. Put the lemon slices on top and drop the butter over. Wrap it up well.

Pour 1 cup of water in and lower the trivet with handle. Put the veggie pack on the trivet, seal the lid, and cook on High Pressure for 2 minutes. Once ready, do a quick release. Carefully remove the packet and serve veggies in a wrap on a plate.

Keto Coconut Almond Cake

Total time: 70 minutes

Ingredients:

1 ½ cups Almond flour

1 cup Shredded Coconut, unsweetened

½ cup Truvia

1 ½ tsp Baking Powder

1 ½ tsp Apple Pie Spice

4 Eggs

½ cup Melted Butter

1 cup Heavy Cream

Directions

Pour all the dry ingredients into a bowl and mix well. Add the wet ingredients one after the other, mixing until fully incorporated. Grease an 8-inch cake tin and pour the batter into it.

Cover the tin with foil and A pinch the edges of the tin to tighten the foil. Pour 2 cups of water into the Instant Pot and fit in a trivet with handles. Place the cake tin on the trivet.

Seal the lid, select Cake mode for 40 minutes on High. Once ready, do a natural pressure release for 10 minutes; then release the remaining pressure. Cool the cake, slice and serve.

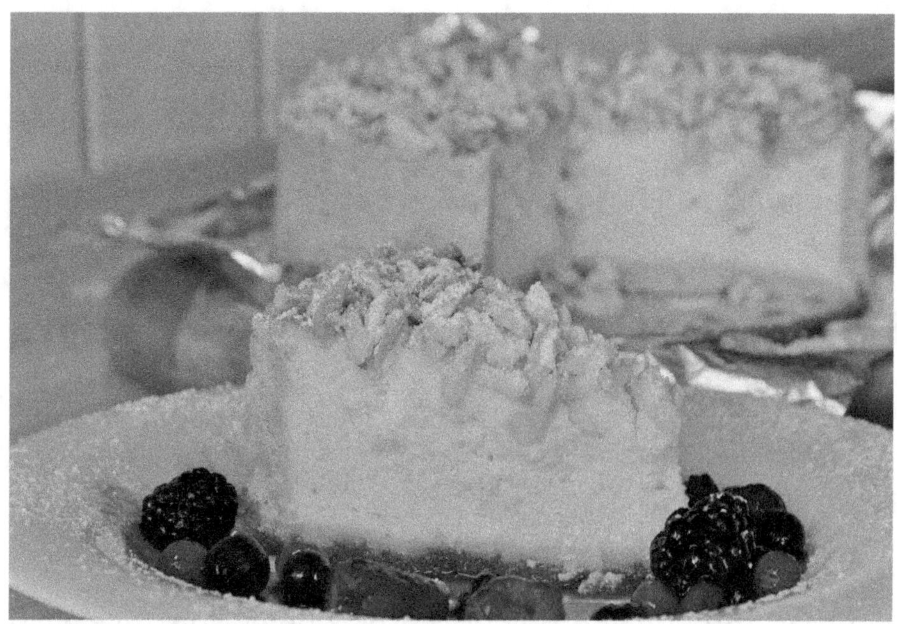

Faux Beet Risotto

Total time: 25 minutes

Ingredients:

4 Beets, tails and leafs removed

2 tbsp Olive oil

1 big head Cauliflower, cut into florets

4 tbsp cup Full Milk

2 tsp Red Chili Flakes

Salt to taste

Black Pepper to taste

½ cup Water

Directions

Pour the water in the Instant Pot and fit a steamer basket. Place the beets and cauliflower in the basket. Seal the lid, and cook on High Pressure mode for 4 minutes.

Once ready, do a natural pressure release for 10 minutes, then quickly release the pressure.Remove the steamer basket with the vegetables and discard water. Remove the beets' peels.

Place veggies back to the pot, add salt, pepper, and flakes. Mash with a potato masher. Hit Sauté, and cook the milk for 2 minutes. Stir frequently. Dish onto plates and drizzle with oil.

Broccoli Rice with Mushrooms

Total time: 40 minutes

Ingredients:

2 tbsp Olive oil

1 small Red Onion, chopped

1 Carrot, chopped

2 cups Button Mushrooms, chopped

½ Lemon, zested and juiced

Salt to taste

Pepper to taste

2 cloves Garlic, minced

½ cup Broccoli rice

½ cup Chicken Stock

5 Cherry Tomatoes

Parsley Leaves, chopped **for garnishing**

Directions

Set on Sauté. Heat oil, and cook the carrots and onions for 2 minutes. Stir in mushrooms, and cook for 3 minutes. Stir in pepper, salt, lemon juice, garlic, and lemon zest.

Stir in broccoli and chicken stock. Drop the tomatoes over the top, but don't stir. Seal the lid, and cook on High pressure for 10 minutes. Once ready, do a natural pressure release for 4 minutes, then quickly release the remaining pressure. Sprinkle with parsley and stir evenly.

Stuffed Cabbages

Total time: 1 hour 45 minutes

Ingredients:

1 medium Cabbage, cut into halves

1 ½ cups Cauliflower, riced

½ lb Ground Beef

¼ Chopped Parsley

2 cloves Garlic, minced

1 Egg, beaten

Salt to taste

Black Pepper to taste

1 tsp Oregano

½ cup Tomato Sauce

¼ cup Sour Cream

1 tbsp Swerve Sweetener

Directions

Pour 1 cup of water in the pot and lower a steamer basket. Place the halves of the cabbage on the basket. Seal the lid, select Manual mode and cook on High pressure for 5 minutes.

Once ready, quickly release the pressure. Remove the cabbage, let it cool and remove as many large leaves off it as possible. Set aside.

In a bowl, add garlic, salt, beef, egg, and cauli rice; mix well. In another bowl, mix the sour cream, tomato sauce, swerve and ¼ cup of water. Pour half of the tomato sauce in a casserole.

Set aside. Lay each cabbage leaf on a flat surface, scoop 2 tbsp of the beef mixture onto each leaf and roll. Arrange the rolls in the casserole dish and pour the remaining tomato sauce over the rolls. Bake it in an oven at 350 F for 1 hour. Flip the cabbages 30 minutes into baking.

Garlic Buttered Sprouts

Total time: 20 minutes

Ingredients:

½ lb Brussels Sprouts, trimmed and washed

½ cup Water

3 tbsp Butter

4 clove Garlic, minced

½ cup Parmesan Cheese, grated

Directions

Pour the water in the Instant Pot and fit a steamer basket. Add the brussels sprouts to the basket. Seal the lid and cook on High Pressure mode for 3 minutes.

Once ready, quickly release the pressure, open the lid and remove the basket. Discard the water and clean dry. Select Sauté, melt the butter and cook the garlic for 1 minute. Add the brussel sprouts; toss evenly. Press Cancel. Serve sprouts and garnish with Parmesan.

Bell Pepper Cream

Total time: 30 minutes

Ingredients:

1 shallot, chopped

2 tablespoons olive oil

4 red bell peppers, roughly chopped

2 tomatoes, cubed

3 tablespoons tomato paste

6 cups chicken stock

½ teaspoon red pepper flakes

1 teaspoon chives, chopped

Directions:

Set the instant pot on Sauté mode, add the oil, heat it up, add the shallot and cook for 2 minutes

Add the rest of the ingredients except the chives, put the lid on and cook on High for 18 minutes.

Release the pressure naturally for 10 minutes, blend the soup using an immersion blender, divide it into bowls and serve.

Chicken and Asparagus Soup

Total time: 30 minutes

Ingredients:

1 asparagus stalk, trimmed and halved

A pinch of salt and black pepper

2 chicken breasts, skinless, boneless and cubed

2 scallions, chopped

1 tablespoon avocado oil

1 tablespoon sweet chili sauce

¼ cup parsley, chopped

5 cups chicken stock

Directions:

Set the instant pot on Sauté mode, add the oil, heat it up, add the scallions and the chili sauce and cook for 3 minutes.

Add the chicken and brown for 2 minutes more.

Add the rest of the ingredients, put the lid on and cook on High for 15 minutes.

Release the pressure naturally for 10 minutes, ladle the soup into bowls and serve.

Hot Cod Stew

Total time: 20 minutes

Ingredients:

1 pound cod fillets, boneless, skinless and cubed

1 cup chicken stock

1 tablespoon hot sauce

1 tablespoon hot paprika

A pinch of salt and black pepper

1 tablespoon cilantro, chopped

Directions:

In your instant pot, combine the cod with the rest of the ingredients, put the lid on and cook on High for 12 minutes.

Release the pressure fast for 5 minutes, divide the stew into bowls and serve.

Lamb Stew

Total time: 40 minutes

Ingredients:

1 tablespoon avocado oil

1 and ½ pound lamb shoulder, cubed

1 cup black olives, pitted and sliced

2 tomatoes, cubed

A pinch of salt and black pepper

1 cup beef stock

1 cup tomato passata

2 tablespoons basil, chopped

Directions:

Set your instant pot on Sauté mode, add the oil, heat it up, add the meat and brown for 5 minutes.

Add the rest of the ingredients except the basil, put the lid on and cook on High for 25 minutes.

Release the pressure naturally for 10 minutes, divide the stew into bowls and serve with the basil, sprinkled on top.

Shrimp and Olives Stew

Total time: 20 minutes

Ingredients:

1 and ½ pounds shrimp, peeled and deveined

1 cup black olives, pitted and halved

2 tablespoons olive oil

2 scallions, chopped

2 tomatoes, cubed

1 tablespoon sweet paprika

½ cup chicken stock

Directions:

Set your instant pot on Sauté mode, add the oil, heat it up, add the scallions and cook for 2 minutes.

Add the rest of the ingredients, put the lid on and cook on Low for 8 minutes.

Release the pressure naturally for 10 minutes, divide the stew into bowls and serve.

Turkey Stew

Total time: 30 minutes

Ingredients:

1 turkey breast, skinless, boneless and cubed

1 teaspoon olive oil

A pinch of salt and black pepper

1 tablespoon avocado oil

1 celery stalk, chopped

2 cups chicken stock

2 cups tomatoes, chopped

1 tablespoons cilantro, chopped

Directions:

Set your instant pot on Sauté mode, add the oil, heat it up, add the meat and cook for 5 minutes.

Add the rest of the ingredients, put the lid on and cook on High for 15 minutes.

Release the pressure naturally for 10 minutes, divide the stew into bowls and serve.

Kale Stew

Total time: 30 minutes

Ingredients:

1 shallot, chopped

2 garlic cloves, minced

1 pound kale, torn

20 ounces canned tomatoes, chopped

2 tablespoons olive oil

A pinch of salt and black pepper

½ teaspoon cayenne pepper

1 tablespoon parsley, chopped

Directions:

Set the instant pot on Sauté mode, add the oil, heat it up, add the shallot and garlic and cook for 2 minutes.

Add the other ingredients, put the lid on and cook on High for 18 minutes.

Release the pressure naturally for 10 minutes, divide the stew into bowls and serve.

Turmeric Cabbage Stew

Total time: 30 minutes

Ingredients:

3 garlic cloves, chopped

1 celery stalk, chopped

2 cups green cabbage, shredded

1 cup veggie stock

½ tablespoon avocado oil

14 ounces canned tomatoes, chopped

A pinch of salt and black pepper

1 teaspoon turmeric powder

Directions:

Set your instant pot on Sauté mode, add the oil, heat it up, add the celery and garlic and sauté for 2 minutes.

Add the rest of the ingredients, put the lid on and cook on High for 15 minutes.

Release the pressure naturally for 10 minutes, divide the stew into bowls and serve.

Chili Mushrooms Stew

Total time: 25 minutes

Ingredients:

2 spring onions, chopped

2 teaspoons avocado oil

2 garlic cloves, minced

1 teaspoon chili powder

A pinch of salt and black pepper

6 cups mushrooms, sliced

2 cups veggie stock

1 cup tomato passata

1 tablespoon chives, chopped

Directions:

Set your instant pot on Sauté mode, add the oil, heat it up, add the onions and the garlic and sauté for 2 minutes.

Add the mushrooms and sauté for 2 minutes more.

Add the rest of the ingredients except the cilantro, put the lid on and cook on High for 10 minutes.

Release the pressure naturally for 10 minutes, divide the stew into bowls and serve with the chives sprinkled on top.

Zucchini and Lamb Stew

Total time: 40 minutes

Ingredients:

2 tablespoons olive oil

2 zucchinis, sliced

A pinch of salt and black pepper

1 pound lamb shoulder, cubed

2 tablespoons tomato passata

¼ cup veggie stock

1 teaspoon sweet paprika

1 tablespoon dill, chopped

Directions:

Set your instant pot on Sauté mode, add the oil, heat it up, the meat and brown for 5 minutes.

Add the rest of the ingredients, put the lid on and cook on High for 25 minutes.

Release the pressure naturally for 10 minutes, divide the stew into bowls and serve.

Chapter 9: Salads Recipes

Salad Wraps

Total time: 30 minutes

Ingredients:

1 tablespoon olive oil

1 teaspoon cumin seeds

1 small yellow onion, thinly sliced

4 cups zucchini, grated

½ teaspoon red pepper flakes, crushed

Salt and ground black pepper, as required

8 large lettuce leaves, rinsed and pat dried

¼ cup Parmesan cheese, shredded

2 tablespoons fresh chives, finely minced

Directions

In a medium skillet, heat the oil over medium-high heat and sauté the cumin seeds for about 1 minute.

Add the onion and sauté for about 4-5 minutes.

Add the zucchini and cook for about 5-7 minutes or until done completely, stirring occasionally.

Stir in the red pepper flakes, salt, and black pepper and remove from the heat.

Arrange the lettuce leaves onto a smooth surface.

Divide the zucchini mixture evenly onto each lettuce leaf.

Top with the Parmesan and fresh chives and serve immediately.

Fresh Veggie Salad

Total time: 30 minutes

Ingredients:

2 cups cucumber, spiralized with blade C

1 cup Kalamata olives, pitted and halved

2 cups grape tomatoes, halved

1 tablespoon fresh oregano, chopped

1 tablespoon fresh basil, chopped

1 garlic clove, minced

2 tablespoons olive oil

2 tablespoons balsamic vinegar

Salt and ground black pepper, as required

Directions

Place all the ingredients in a large serving bowl and toss to coat well.

Serve immediately.

Berries & Spinach Salad

Total time: 20 minutes

Ingredients:

For Salad:

8 ounces fresh baby spinach

¾ cup fresh strawberries, hulled and sliced

¾ cup fresh blueberries

¼ cup feta cheese, crumbled

 For Dressing:

1/3 cup olive oil

2 tablespoons fresh lemon juice

¼ teaspoon liquid stevia

1/8 teaspoon paprika

1/8 teaspoon garlic powder

Salt, as required

Directions

For salad: in a bowl, mix together the spinach, berries and almonds.

For dressing: in another small bowl, add all the ingredients and beat until well combined.

Place the dressing over salad and gently, toss to coat well.

Serve immediately.

Cabbage Salad

Total time: 20 minutes

Ingredients:

For Salad:

4 cups green cabbage, shredded

¼ onion, thinly sliced

1 teaspoon lime zest, grated freshly

3 tablespoons fresh cilantro, chopped

 For Dressing:

¾ cup mayonnaise

2 teaspoons fresh lime juice

2 teaspoons chili sauce

½ teaspoon Erythritol

2 garlic cloves, minced

Directions

For salad: in a bowl, mix together the cabbage, onion, lime zest and cilantro.

For dressing: in another small bowl, add all the ingredients and beat until well combined.

Place the dressing over salad and gently, toss to coat well.

Cover and refrigerate to chill before serving.

Cucumber & Spinach Salad

Total time: 20 minutes

Ingredients:

For Dressing:

5 tablespoons olive oil

4 tablespoons plain Greek yogurt

2 tablespoons fresh lemon juice

2 tablespoons fresh mint leaves, finely chopped

1 teaspoon Erythritol

Salt and ground black pepper, as required

For Salad:

3 cups cucumbers, peeled, seeded and sliced

10 cups fresh baby spinach

¼ of medium yellow onion, sliced

Directions

For dressing: add all the ingredients in a bowl and beat until well combined.

Cover and refrigerate to chill for about 1 hour.

In a large serving bowl, mix together all the salad ingredients.

Place dressing over salad and toss to coat well.

Serve immediately.

Broccoli Salad

Total time: 20 minutes

Ingredients:

For Salad:

8 cups small fresh broccoli florets

1 (8-ounces) package Colby-Monterey Jack cheese, cubed

2 cups fresh strawberries, hulled and sliced

¼ cup fresh mint leaves, chopped

 For Dressing:

1 cup mayonnaise

1 teaspoon balsamic vinegar

2 teaspoons Erythritol

Salt and ground black pepper, as required

Directions

For salad: in a large serving bowl, add all the ingredients and mix well.

For the dressing: in another bowl, add all the ingredients and beat until well combined.

Place the dressing over salad and gently, stir to combine.

Serve immediately.

Tomato & Mozzarella Salad

Total time: 20 minutes

Ingredients:

4 cups cherry tomatoes, halved

1½ pounds mozzarella cheese, cubed

¼ cup fresh basil leaves, chopped

¼ cup olive oil

2 tablespoons fresh lemon juice

1 teaspoon fresh oregano, minced

1 teaspoon fresh parsley, minced

2-4 drops liquid stevia

Salt and ground black pepper, as required

Directions

In a salad bowl, mix together the tomatoes, mozzarella and basil.

In another small bowl, place the remaining ingredients and beat until well combined.

Place dressing over salad and toss to coat well.

Serve immediately.

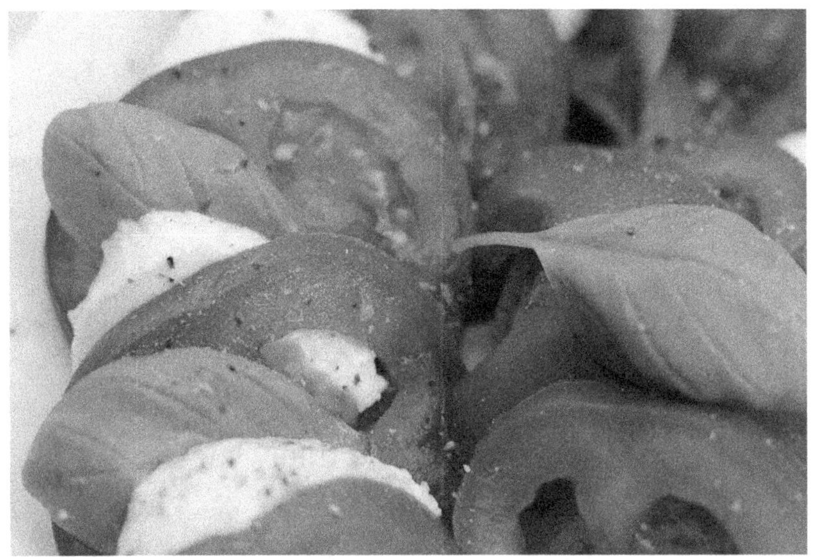

Mixed Veggie Salad

Total time: 25 minutes

Ingredients:

For Dressing:

1 small avocado, peeled, pitted and chopped

¼ cup plain Greek yogurt

1 small yellow onion, chopped

1 garlic clove, chopped

2 tablespoons fresh parsley

2 tablespoons fresh lemon juice

For Salad:

6 cups fresh spinach, shredded

2 medium zucchinis, cut into thin slices

½ cup celery, sliced

½ cup red bell pepper, seeded and thinly sliced

½ cup yellow onion, thinly sliced

½ cup cucumber, thinly sliced

½ cup cherry tomatoes, halved

¼ cup Kalamata olives, pitted

½ cup feta cheese, crumbled

Directions

For dressing: in a food processor, add all the ingredients and pulse until smooth.

For the salad: in a salad bowl, add all the ingredients and mix well.

Place the dressing over salad and gently, toss to coat well.

Serve immediately.

Creamy Shrimp Salad

 Total time: 23 minutes

Ingredients:

4 pounds large shrimp

1 lemon, quartered

3 cups celery stalks, chopped

1 yellow onion, chopped

2 cups mayonnaise

2 tablespoons fresh lemon juice

1 teaspoon Dijon mustard

Salt and ground black pepper, as required

Directions

In a pan of lightly salted boiling water, add the shrimp, and lemon and cook for about 3 minutes.

Drain the shrimps well and let them cool.

Then, peel and devein the shrimps.

In a large bowl, add the cooked shrimp and remaining ingredients and gently, stir to combine.

Serve immediately.

Shrimp & Green Beans Salad

Total time: 28 minutes

Ingredients:

For Shrimp:

2 tablespoons olive oil

2 tablespoons fresh key lime juice

4 large garlic cloves, peeled

2 sprigs fresh rosemary leaves

½ teaspoon garlic salt

20 large shrimp, peeled and deveined

For Salad:

1 pound fresh green beans, trimmed

¼ cup olive oil

1 onion, sliced

Salt and ground black pepper, as required

½ cup garlic and herb feta cheese, crumbled

Directions

For shrimp marinade: in a blender, add all the ingredients except shrimp and pulse until smooth.

Transfer the marinade in a large bowl.

Place the shrimp and generously mix with marinade.

Cover the bowl and refrigerate to marinate for at least 30 minutes.

Preheat the broiler of oven. Arrange the rack in top position of oven. Line a large baking sheet with a piece of foil.

Place shrimp with marinade onto the prepared baking sheet.

Broil for about 3-4 minutes per side.

Transfer the shrimp mixture into a bowl and refrigerate until using.

Meanwhile, for the salad: in a pan of salted boiling water, add the green beans and cook for about 3-4 minutes.

Drain the green beans well and rinse under cold running water.

Transfer the green beans into a large bowl.

Add the oil, onion, shrimp, salt and black pepper and stir to combine.

Cover and refrigerate to chill for about 1 hour.

Stir in the cheese just before serving.

Salmon Salad

Total time: 20 minutes

Ingredients:

12 hard-boiled organic eggs, peeled and cubed

1 pound smoked salmon, chopped

3 celery stalks, chopped

1 yellow onion, chopped

4 tablespoons fresh dill, chopped

2 cups mayonnaise

Salt and ground black pepper, as required

8 cups fresh lettuce leaves

Directions

In a large serving bowl, add all the ingredients except lettuce leaves and gently stir to combine.

Cover and refrigerate to chill before serving.

Divide the lettuce onto serving plates and top with salmon salad.

Serve immediately.

Lobster Salad

Total time: 20 minutes

Ingredients:

5 pounds cooked lobster meat, shredded

3 yellow bell peppers, seeded and chopped

6 celery stalks, chopped

1 large yellow onion, chopped

2 cups mayonnaise

Freshly ground black pepper, as required

Directions

In a salad bowl, add all the ingredients and mix until well combined.

Refrigerate to chill before serving.

Tuna Salad

Total time: 25 minutes

Ingredients:

2 (6-ounces) cans water packed solid white tuna, drained

¼ cup fresh cranberries

3 tablespoons mayonnaise

1/3 teaspoon dried dill weed

Directions

In a large salad bowl, place the tuna and with a fork, mash it completely.

Add the remaining ingredients and stir to mix well.

Serve immediately.

Crab Salad

Total time: 20 minutes

Ingredients:

1 pound jumbo lump crabmeat, picked over

1 celery stalk, peeled, and cut into 1/8-inch pieces

4 teaspoons fresh chives, minced

1 teaspoon fresh tarragon leaves, minced

1/3 cup mayonnaise

2 tablespoons sour cream

1 teaspoon fresh lemon juice

½ teaspoon Dijon mustard

Salt and ground black pepper, as required

Directions

In a bowl, add the crabmeat, celery, chives, and tarragon and toss to coat well.

In another bowl, mix well mayonnaise, sour cream, lemon juice, mustard, salt and black pepper.

Place the dressing into bowl of crabmeat mixture and gently, stir to combine.

Serve immediately.

Beef Salad

Total time: 225 minutes

Ingredients:

1 pound grass-fed ground beef

1 teaspoon olive oil

1 tablespoon taco seasoning

8 ounces Romaine lettuce, chopped

1 1/3 cups grape tomatoes, halved

1 large cucumber, chopped

½ cup scallions, chopped

¾ cup Cheddar cheese, shredded

1/3 cup salsa

1/3 cup sour cream

Directions

In a skillet, heat the oil over high heat and stir fry beef for about 8-10 minutes, breaking up the beef with a spatula.

Stir in the taco seasoning and remove from heat.

Set aside to cool slightly.

Meanwhile, in a large bowl, add the remaining ingredients and mix until well combined.

Add the ground beef and toss to coat well.

Serve immediately.

Turkey Salad

Total time: 33 minutes

Ingredients:

1 pound ground turkey

1 tablespoon olive oil

Salt and ground black pepper, as required

¼ cup water

½ of English cucumber, chopped

4 cups green cabbage, shredded

½ cup fresh mint leaves, chopped

2 tablespoons fresh lime juice

¼ cup walnuts, chopped

Directions

Heat the oil in a skillet over medium-high heat and cook the turkey for about 6-8 minutes, breaking up the meat with a spatula.

Stir in the salt, black pepper, and water and cook for about 4-5 minutes or until almost all the liquid is evaporated.

Remove from heat and transfer the turkey into a bowl.

Set the bowl aside to cool completely.

In a large serving bowl, mix well vegetables, mint and lime juice.

Add the cooked turkey and stir to combine.

Top with the chopped walnuts and serve.

Chicken Salad

Total time: 36 minutes

Ingredients:

2 pounds grass-fed boneless, skinless chicken breasts

½ cup olive oil

¼ cup fresh lemon juice

2 tablespoons Erythritol

1 garlic clove, minced

Salt and ground black pepper, as required

4 cups fresh strawberries, hulled and sliced

8 cups fresh spinach, torn

Directions

For marinade: in a large bowl, add the oil, lemon juice, Erythritol, garlic, salt, and black pepper and beat until well combined.

Place chicken and ¾ cup marinade in a large resealable plastic bag.

Seal bag and shake to coat well.

Refrigerate overnight.

Cover the bowl of remaining marinade and refrigerate before serving.

Preheat the grill to medium heat. Grease the grill grate.

Remove the chicken from bag and discard the marinade.

Place the chicken onto grill grate and grill, covered for about 5-8 minutes per side.

Remove the chicken from grill and cut into bite sized pieces.

In a large bowl, mix together the chicken pieces, strawberries and spinach.

Add the reserved marinade and toss to coat.

Serve immediately.

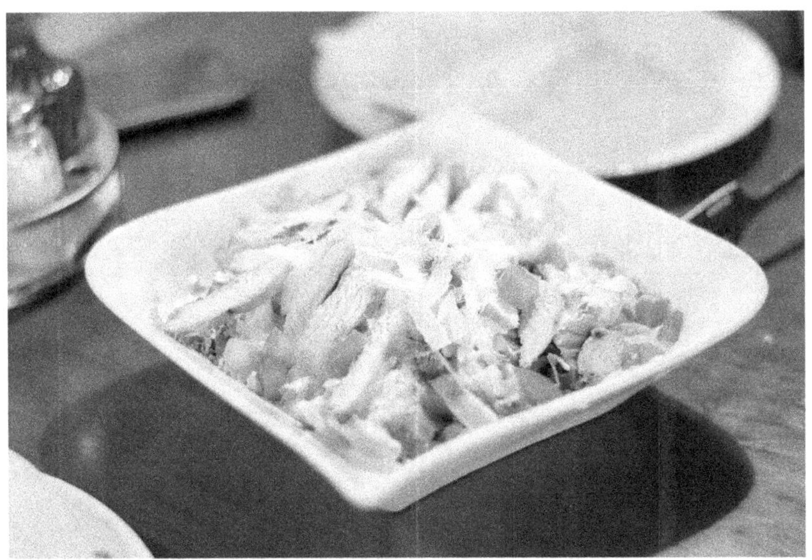

Chapter 10: Soup Recipes

Creamy Kale Soup

Total time: 15 minutes

Ingredients:

4 stalks celery, trimmed and chopped

8 cloves garlic, peeled and minced

1 tablespoon butter

1 package (16 ouncesfrozen chopped kale

1 package (16 ouncesfrozen cauliflower florets

4 cups beef or chicken stock

1 tablespoon balsamic vinegar

Salt and freshly ground pepper, to taste

½ cup heavy cream

4 tablespoons finely grated Parmesan cheese

1 onion, diced

Directions

In Instant Pot on sauté setting, cook onion, celery and garlic in butter until slightly softened, about 2 minutes.

Add kale, cauliflower, stock and balsamic vinegar to pot and season to taste with salt and pepper.

Secure pot lid, close pressure valve and cook on high for 3 minutes. Let pressure release naturally.

Slowly pour cream into soup, stirring constantly. Mash some of the cauliflower if desired for a thicker consistency.

Ladle soup into bowls and garnish with Parmesan cheese to serve.

Enjoy!

Broccoli Cheese Soup

Total time: 30 minutes

Ingredients:

2 tablespoons butter

1 medium onion, diced

4 cloves garlic, peeled and minced

4 cups chicken stock

4 cups broccoli florets

1 cup heavy cream

8 ounces Colby cheese, shredded

Directions

In Instant Pot on sauté setting, melt butter and cook onion and garlic until translucent, about 5 minutes.

Add broccoli and chicken stock to pot and season to taste with salt and pepper. Secure pot lid, close pressure valve and cook on high setting for 5 minutes.

When cooking time ends, carefully turn venting knob from sealing to venting position for a quick pressure release.

Add heavy cream and Colby cheese to soup and stir until cheese is melted.

Season soup to taste with salt and pepper, serve and enjoy!

Broccoli Cauliflower Soup

Total time: 45 minutes

Ingredients:

1 small onion, diced

3 cloves garlic, peeled and minced

1 package (10 ouncesfrozen broccoli

1 package (10 ouncesfrozen cauliflower

4 cups chicken stock

1 package (3 ouncescream cheese, softened

¼ teaspoon ground nutmeg

6 ounces sharp cheddar cheese, shredded

Salt and freshly ground black pepper, to taste

1 tablespoon butter stalks celery, trimmed and diced

Directions

In Instant Pot on sauté setting, melt butter and cook celery, onion and garlic until translucent, about 5 minutes.

Add broccoli, cauliflower, chicken stock, cream cheese and nutmeg to pot and season to taste with salt and pepper.

Secure pot lid, close pressure valve and cook on high setting for 30 minutes. When cooking time ends, let pressure release naturally.

For chunky soup, serve immediately; otherwise puree soup with an immersion blender to desired texture.

Garnish servings of soup with grated cheese and enjoy!

Clam and Cauliflower Chowder

Total time: 25 minutes

Ingredients:

3 (6.5-ouncecans chopped clams

3 tablespoons butter

1 small yellow onion

4 cups chopped cauliflower

1 ½ cups heavy cream

½ teaspoon dried thyme

Salt and pepper

Directions:

Drain the clams into a bowl and add water to the juice to make 2 cups of liquid.

Turn the Instant Pot on to the Sauté setting then add the butter and onion.

Cook for 2 minutes then add the cauliflower and clam juice.

Close and lock the lid then push the Manual button and set the timer for 5 minutes.

When the timer goes off, let the pressure vent for 3 minutes then press Cancel and do a Quick Release by switching the steam valve to "venting". When the pot has depressurized, stir in the clams and heavy cream.

Cook on the Sauté setting until heated through then season with thyme, salt, and pepper. Serve hot.

Turkey Soup

Total time: 35 minutes

Ingredients:

1 medium red bell pepper, diced

4 stalks celery, trimmed and diced

2 cloves garlic, peeled and minced

2 tablespoons butter

1-pound boneless skinless turkey thighs

Salt and freshly ground black pepper, to taste

½ teaspoon dried thyme

1 large bay leaf

2 small zucchinis, diced

1 cup frozen peas

1 tablespoon fresh cilantro, minced

½ teaspoon dried basil

1 onion, diced

4 cups chicken stock ½ teaspoon dried oregano

Directions

In Instant Pot on sauté setting, cook onion, bell pepper, celery and garlic in butter until onion is translucent, about 5 minutes. Move onion mixture to sides of pot.

Season turkey thighs to taste with salt and pepper, add to pot and cook on both sides until lightly browned, 2-3 minutes per side.

Add chicken stock, oregano, basil, thyme and bay leaf to pot and season soup to taste with salt and pepper.

Secure pot lid, close pressure valve and cook on high setting for 15 minutes. When cooking time ends, carefully turn venting knob from sealing to venting position for a quick pressure release.

Remove turkey thighs from pot and dice or shred as desired. Return turkey to pot and add zucchini and peas.

Cover pot and let soup stand until zucchini and peas are warmed, about 5 minutes. Remove bay leaf from soup.

Ladle soup into bowls and garnish with cilantro.

Serve and enjoy!

Buffalo Chicken Soup

Total time: 20 minutes

Ingredients:

1 tablespoon olive oil

½ cup diced yellow onion

1-pound boneless chicken thighs, chopped (cooked

4 cups chicken broth

3 tablespoons hot sauce

6 ounces cream cheese, chopped

½ cup heavy cream

Directions:

Turn the Instant Pot on to the Sauté setting and let it heat up.

Add the oil then stir in the onion and cook for 3 to 4 minutes. Stir in the chicken, chicken broth, and hot sauce.

Close and lock the lid then press the Soup button and adjust the timer to 5 minutes. When the timer goes off, let the pressure vent for 5 minutes then do a Quick Release by pressing the Cancel button and switching the steam valve to "venting". When the pot has depressurized, open the lid.

Spoon a cup of the soup into a blender and add the cream cheese. Blend smooth then stir the mixture back into the pot with the heavy cream.

Stir until smooth then serve hot.

Ham & Asparagus Soup

Total time: 85 minutes

Ingredients:

1 onion, diced

4 stalks celery, trimmed and diced

2 cloves garlic, peeled and minced

1 meaty ham bone

4 cups chicken stock

2 pounds asparagus stalks

1 bay leaf

½ teaspoon dried thyme

Salt and ground black pepper, to taste

1 tablespoon butter

Directions

Melt butter in instant pot on sauté setting and cook onion, celery and garlic until softened, about 5 minutes.

Add ham bone and stock to pot and simmer for 3 minutes.

Peel and trim asparagus stalks as necessary, cut in half and add to pot with thyme. Season soup to taste with salt and pepper.

Secure pot lid, close pressure valve and cook on soup setting for about 45 minutes. When cooking time ends, let pressure release naturally.

Remove ham bone and shred ham with a fork. If desired, blend soup with an immersion blender to desired consistency.

Stir ham into soup, serve and enjoy!

Hearty Beef and Bacon Chili

Total time: 45 minutes

Ingredients:

6 slices bacon, chopped

2 small red peppers, chopped

1-pound ground beef (80% lean

1 cup diced tomatoes

1 cup low-carb tomato sauce

2 tablespoons chili powder

1 teaspoon garlic powder

Salt and pepper

Directions:

Turn on the Instant Pot to the Sauté setting and add the chopped bacon. Let the bacon cook until it is crisp then remove it with a slotted spoon.

Add the red peppers to the pot. Cook for 5 minutes, stirring, then add the rest of the ingredients.

Close and lock the lid then press the Bean/Chili button to cook for 30 minutes. When the timer goes off, let the pressure vent for 10 minutes then press Cancel to do a Quick Release by switching the steam valve to "venting".

Open the lid when the pot has depressurized and stir in the bacon.

Season with salt and pepper to taste then serve hot.

Chicken Tomato Sausage Stew

Total time: 30 minutes

Ingredients:

1 tablespoon coconut oil

1-pound Andouille pork sausage

1 medium white onion, thinly sliced

6 cups tomatoes, chopped

4-pound chicken thighs, boneless, skinless

3 bell peppers, diced

2 celery stalks, chopped

2 cups water or bone broth

2 large carrots, chopped

6 garlic cloves, minced

/4 cup parsley, minced

1 teaspoon thyme

1 teaspoon salt

1/2 teaspoon red chili flakes, crushed

1/2 teaspoon smoked paprika

1/4 teaspoon cayenne

1/4 teaspoon black pepper hot sauce (if desired

1 bay leaf

Directions

Put coconut oil into Instant Pot. Press "Sauté" button, put sausage and chicken into Instant Pot and sauté till the meat is evenly cooked. Take out cooked meat and set aside.

Put celery, onions, bell peppers, and carrots into Instant Pot.

Press "Sauté" button and stir from time to time.

Put minced garlic into Instant Pot and continue sautéing.

Put chopped tomatoes and broth into Instant Pot.

Continue sautéing until simmering.

Once cooled, slice sausage and chicken into small chunks.

Put sausage, chicken, spices and the minced parsley into Instant Pot, stir until evenly mixed.

Close the lid, and turn the vent to "Sealed".

Press "Soup" button, set the timer for 5-10 minutes and set "Pressure" to high.

Once the timer is up press "Cancel" button and turn the steam release handle to "Venting" position for quick release, until the float valve drops down.

Open the lid.

Serve warm, topped with hot sauce (if desired.

Green Beans Soup

Total time: 30 minutes

Ingredients:

2 tablespoons olive oil

1 shallot, chopped

1 teaspoon garlic, minced

1 red bell pepper, chopped

8 cups chicken stock

1 and ½ pounds green beans, trimmed and halved

1 cup tomatoes, chopped

1 tablespoon chili powder

1 cup coconut cream

Directions:

Set your instant pot on sauté mode, add the oil, heat it up, add the shallot and the garlic and sauté for 2 minutes.

Add the rest of the ingredients, put the lid on and cook on High for 13 minutes.

Release the pressure naturally for 10 minutes, divide the soup into bowls and serve.

Bay Leaves Carrots Kale Chicken Soup

Total time: 14 minutes

Ingredients:

2 tablespoons olive oil or butter

3 carrots, peeled & cut into small bite-sized pieces

1 medium onion, chopped

2 bay leaves

4 celery stalks, cut into small bite-sized pieces

1/2 teaspoon black pepper

1 teaspoon salt

1/4 teaspoon oregano, dried

1/2 teaspoon thyme, dried

1-pound chicken breast, cooked, shredded

4 cups chicken broth + 1 cup water

1/2 teaspoon Worcestershire sauce or fish sauce

1 cup kale, chopped

Directions

Put butter or oil into Instant Pot. Press "Sauté" and add onions. Sauté for 5 minutes with the lid open, until soft.

Add oregano, thyme, pepper, salt, bay leaves, celery and carrots into Instant Pot. Keep sautéing for 1 more minute, until fragrant.

Add water and broth into Instant Pot. Close the lid and turn the vent to "Sealed".

Press "Soup", set the timer for 4 minutes and set "Pressure" to high. Once the timer is up press "Cancel" button and turn the steam release handle to "Venting" position for quick release, until the float valve drops down.

Open the lid.

Add kale and chicken into Instant Pot and let sit for 1 minute until kale turns bright green.

Add pepper, salt and fish sauce and stir to incorporate.

Broccoli and Zucchini Soup

Total time: 30 minutes

Ingredients:

1 shallot, chopped

2 teaspoons avocado oil

1-pound broccoli florets

1-pound zucchinis, sliced

4 cups chicken stock

1 teaspoon basil, dried

1 tablespoon cilantro, chopped

Directions:

Set your instant pot on sauté mode, add the oil, heat it up, add the shallot and sauté for 2 minutes.

Add the broccoli and the rest of the ingredients, put the lid on and cook on High for 12 minutes.

Release the pressure naturally for 10 minutes, ladle the soup into bowls and serve.

Healthy Creamy Mushroom Stew

Total time: 45 minutes

Ingredients:

1 celery stalk, chopped

2 Tablespoons green onions, chopped

2 garlic cloves, minced

2 cups beef stock

½ cup heavy cream

5 ounces cream cheese, softened

1 Tablespoon unsalted butter, melted

1 Tablespoon lemon juice

1 teaspoon fresh or dried thyme

2 Tablespoons fresh sage, chopped

1 bay leaf

1 teaspoon salt

1-pound cremini mushrooms, sliced

1 teaspoon fresh ground black pepper

Directions

Rinse the mushrooms, pat dry.

Press Sauté button on Instant Pot and melt the butter.

Add green onions, garlic. Cook for 1 minute.

Add mushrooms, celery, and garlic. Sauté until vegetables are softened.

Press Keep Warm/Cancel setting to stop Sauté mode.

Add remaining ingredients. Stir well.

Close and seal lid. Select Meat/Stew button. Set cooking time to 20 minutes. Once done, Instant Pot will switch to Keep Warm mode.

Remain on Keep Warm for 10 minutes.

When done, use Quick Release setting; turn valve from sealing to venting to release pressure quickly. Open lid carefully.

Stir ingredients and serve.

Garnish with green onion, grated parmesan cheese.

Beef Soup

Total time: 40 minutes

Ingredients:

A pinch of salt and black pepper

1 and ½ pound beef meat, cubed

1 cup scallions, chopped

2 tablespoons olive oil

1 tablespoon sweet paprika

6 cups veggie stock

1 tablespoon parsley, chopped

Directions:

Set your instant pot on sauté mode, add the oil, heat it up, add the meat and the scallions and brown for 5 minutes.

Add the rest of the ingredients, put the lid on and cook on High for 20 minutes.

Release the pressure naturally for 10 minutes, ladle the soup into bowls and serve

Creamy Artichoke Spinach Soup

Total time: 30 minutes

Ingredients:

4 cups spinach

1-ounce jar artichoke hearts, drained and chopped

4 cups low-sodium chicken broth

¼ cup cheddar cheese, shredded

¼ cup mozzarella cheese, shredded

1 Tablespoon butter, melted

1 Tablespoon Italian seasoning

2 teaspoons fresh parsley, chopped

1 teaspoon salt

1 bunch of kale, stemmed and chopped

1 teaspoon fresh ground black pepper

Directions

Place all ingredients in Instant Pot. Stir well.

Close and seal lid. Press Manual setting. Cook for 15 minutes.

When done, use Quick-Release setting. Open lid carefully. Stir ingredients.

Serve.

Spinach Soup

Total time: 35 minutes

Ingredients:

2 teaspoons olive oil

scallion, chopped

1 celery stalk, chopped

4 cups baby spinach

4 garlic cloves, minced

teaspoons cumin, ground

6 cups veggie stock

1 teaspoon basil, dried

Directions:

Set your instant pot on sauté mode, add the oil, heat it up, add the scallion and garlic and sauté for 5 minutes.

Add the celery, cumin and the basil and sauté for 4 minutes more.

Add the spinach and the stock, put the lid on and cook on High for 10 minutes.

4.Release the pressure naturally for 10 minutes, ladle the soup into bowls and serve.

Cilantro Avocado Chicken Soup

Total time: 45 minutes

Ingredients:

4 chicken breasts, boneless, skinless

1 tablespoon coconut oil

4 avocados, peeled and chopped

4 cups chicken broth

Zest and juice from 1 lime

1 Tablespoon fresh cilantro, chopped

1 teaspoon salt

1 teaspoon fresh ground black pepper

2 tomatoes, chopped

2 garlic cloves, minced

Directions

Rinse the chicken, pat dry. Cut into strips.

Press Sauté button on Instant Pot. Melt the coconut oil.

Add chicken strips. Sauté until chicken no longer pink.

Add garlic and tomatoes. Stir well.

Press Keep Warm/Cancel setting to stop Sauté mode.

Add chopped avocados, chicken broth, lime juice, lime zest, cilantro, salt, and black pepper. Stir well.

Close and seal lid. Press Meat/Stew button on Instant Pot. Cook for 20 minutes.

Once done, Instant Pot will switch to Keep Warm mode.

Remain in Keep Warm mode for 10 minutes.

When done, use Quick-Release. Open lid carefully. Stir ingredients. Serve.

Broccoli Coconut Beef Curry Stew

Total time: 55 minutes

Ingredients:

2 1/2-pound beef stew chunks, chopped into small cubes

3 zucchinis, chopped

1-pound broccoli florets

2 tablespoons curry powder

½ cup water or chicken broth

1 tablespoon garlic power

14 oz. can coconut milk

salt to taste

Directions

Put every ingredient into Instant Pot, and stir until evenly mixed.

Close the lid, and turn the vent to "Sealed"

Press "Manual" button, set the timer for 45 minutes and set "Pressure" to high.

Once the timer is up press "Cancel" button and turn the steam release handle to "Venting" position for quick release, until the float valve drops down.

Open the lid.

Add coconut milk and stir with a wooden spoon until evenly mixed. Salt to taste.

Chapter 11: Snacks Recipes

Chicken Popcorns

(Total time: 40 minutes

Ingredients:

½ pound grass-fed chicken thigh, cut into bite-sized pieces

7 ounces unsweetened coconut milk

1 teaspoon ground turmeric

Salt and ground black pepper, as required

2 tablespoons coconut flour

3 tablespoons desiccated coconut

1 tablespoon coconut oil, melted

Directions

Place the chicken, coconut milk, turmeric, salt and black pepper in a large bowl and mix well.

Cover the bowl and refrigerate to marinate overnight.

Preheat the oven to 390 degrees F.

Place the coconut flour and desiccated coconut in a shallow dish and mix well.

Coat the chicken pieces evenly with coconut mixture.

Arrange the chicken piece onto a baking sheet and drizzle with oil.

Bake for about 20-25 minutes.

Remove the baking sheet from oven and transfer the chicken popcorn onto a platter.

Set aside to cool slightly.

Serve warm.

Chicken Nuggets

Total time: 45 minutes

Ingredients:

2 (8-ounces) grass-fed skinless, boneless chicken breasts, cut into 2x1-inch chunks

2 organic eggs

1 cup almond flour

1 teaspoon dried oregano, crushed

½ teaspoon onion powder

½ teaspoon garlic powder

½ teaspoon paprika

Salt and ground black pepper, as required

Directions

Preheat the oven to 350 degrees F. Grease a baking sheet.

Crack the eggs in a shallow bowl and beat well.

Place the flour, oregano, spices, salt, and black pepper in another shallow bowl and mix until well combined.

Dip the chicken nuggets in beaten eggs and then, evenly coat with the flour mixture.

Arrange the chicken nuggets onto prepared baking sheet in a single layer.

Bake for about 30 minutes or until golden brown.

Remove from the oven and set aside to cool slightly.

Serve warm.

Tuna Croquettes

Total time: 31 minutes

Ingredients:

24 ounces canned white tuna, drained

¼ cup mayonnaise

4 large organic eggs

2 tablespoons yellow onion, finely chopped

1 scallion, thinly sliced

4 garlic cloves, minced

¾ cup almond flour

Salt and ground black pepper, as required

¼ cup olive oil

Directions

Place the tuna, mayonnaise, eggs, onion, scallion, garlic, almond flour, salt, and black pepper in a large bowl and mix until well combined.

Make 8 equal-sized oblong shaped patties from the mixture.

Heat the olive oil in a large skillet over medium-high heat and fry the croquettes in 2 batches for about 2-4 minutes per side.

With a slotted spoon, transfer the croquettes onto a paper towel-lined plate to drain completely.

Serve warm.

Brussels Sprout Chips

Total time: 35 minutes

Ingredients:

½ pound Brussels sprouts, thinly sliced

4 tablespoons Parmesan cheese, grated and divided

1 tablespoon olive oil

1 teaspoon garlic powder

Salt and ground black pepper, as required

Directions

Preheat the oven to 400 degrees F. Lightly grease a large baking sheet.

Place the Brussels sprout slices, 2 tablespoons of Parmesan cheese, oil, garlic powder, salt, and black pepper in a large mixing bowl and toss to coat well.

Arrange the Brussels sprout slices onto prepared baking sheet in an even layer.

Bake for about 18-20 minutes, tossing once halfway through.

Remove from oven and transfer the Brussels sprout chips onto a platter.

Sprinkle with the remaining cheese and serve.

Cauliflower Popcorns

Total time: 45 minutes

Ingredients:

4 cups large cauliflower florets

2 teaspoons butter, melted

Salt, as required

3 tablespoons Parmesan cheese, shredded

Directions

Preheat the oven to 450 degrees F. Grease a roasting pan.

Add all the ingredients except Parmesan in a large bowl and toss to coat well.

Place the cauliflower florets into prepared roasting pan and spread in an even layer.

Roast for about 25-30 minutes.

Remove from oven and transfer the cauliflower popcorns onto a platter.

Sprinkle with the Parmesan cheese and serve.

3 Cheese Crackers

Total time: 34 minutes

Ingredients:

2 ounces cream cheese

1 cup Parmesan cheese, grated

1 cup Romano cheese, grated

1 cup almond flour

1 organic egg

1 teaspoon dried rosemary

¼ teaspoon Cajun seasoning

Salt, as required

Directions

Preheat the oven to 450 degrees F and line a baking sheet with parchment paper.

Place the cream cheese, Parmesan cheese, Romano cheese, and almond flour in a microwave-safe bowl and microwave on High for about 1 minute, stirring once halfway through.

Remove from microwave and immediately, stir the mixture until well combined.

Set aside to cool for about 2-3 minutes.

In the same bowl of cheese mixture, add the egg, rosemary, seasoning, and salt and mix until a dough forms.

Arrange the dough between 2 large parchment papers and place onto a smooth surface.

With a lightly floured rolling pin, roll the dough into a thin layer.

Remove the upper parchment paper and with a knife, cut the dough into desired-sized crackers.

Carefully, arrange the crackers onto prepared baking sheet in a single layer about 1-inch apart.

Bake for about 6-7 minutes per side or until crispy.

Remove from oven and let the crackers cool completely before serving.

Enjoy!

Cheese Bites

Total time: 20 minutes

Ingredients:

8 ounces provolone cheese, shredded

½ teaspoon paprika

Directions

Preheat the oven to 400 degrees F and line a baking sheet with parchment paper.

With a spoon, place the cheese in small heaps onto the prepared baking sheet, leaving about 1-inch apart.

Sprinkle evenly with paprika and bake for about 8-10 minutes.

Remove from oven and let the chips cool completely before serving.

Serve.

Cheese Chips

Total time: 30 minutes

Ingredients:

3 tablespoons coconut flour

½ cup strong cheddar cheese, grated and divided

¼ cup Parmesan cheese, grated

2 tablespoons butter, melted

1 organic egg

1 teaspoon fresh thyme leaves, minced

Directions

Preheat the oven to 350 degrees F and line a baking sheet with parchment paper.

Place the coconut flour, ¼ cup of grated cheddar, Parmesan, butter, and egg and mix until well combined.

Set the mixture aside for about 3-5 minutes.

Make 8 equal-sized balls from the mixture.

Arrange the balls onto prepared baking sheet in a single layer about 2-inch apart.

With your hands, press each ball into a little flat disc.

Sprinkle each disc with the remaining cheddar, followed by thyme.

Bake for about 13-15 minutes or until the edges become golden brown.

Remove from the oven and let them cool completely before serving.

Serve.

Cheddar Biscuits

 Total time: 30 minutes

Ingredients:

1/3 cup coconut flour, sifted

¼ teaspoon organic baking powder

Salt, as required

4 organic eggs

¼ cup butter, melted and cooled

1 cup cheddar cheese, shredded

Directions

Preheat the oven to 400 degrees F and line a large cookie sheet with a greased piece of foil.

In a large bowl, add the flour, baking powder, and salt and mix until well combined.

In another bowl, add the eggs and butter and beat until smooth.

Add egg mixture into the bowl of flour mixture and beat until well combined.

Fold in the cheddar cheese.

With a tablespoon, place the mixture onto prepared cookie sheet in a single layer and with your fingers, press slightly.

Bake for 15 minutes or until top becomes golden brown.

Remove the cookie sheet from oven and place onto a wire rack to cool for about 5 minutes.

Carefully, invert the biscuits onto wire rack to cool completely before serving.

Serve.

Cinnamon Cookies

Total time: 40 minutes

Ingredients:

2 cups almond meal

1 teaspoon ground cinnamon

1 organic egg

½ cup salted butter, softened

1 teaspoon liquid stevia

1 teaspoon organic vanilla extract

Directions

Preheat the oven to 300 degrees F and grease a large cookie sheet.

Place all the ingredients in a large bowl and mix until well combined.

Make 15 equal-sized balls from the mixture.

Arrange the balls onto prepared baking sheet about 2-inch apart.

Bake for about 5 minutes.

Remove the cookies from oven and with a fork, press down each ball.

Bake or about another 18-20 minutes.

Remove from oven and place the cookie sheet onto a wire rack to cool for about 5 minutes.

Carefully, invert the cookies onto the wire rack to cool completely before serving.

Serve.

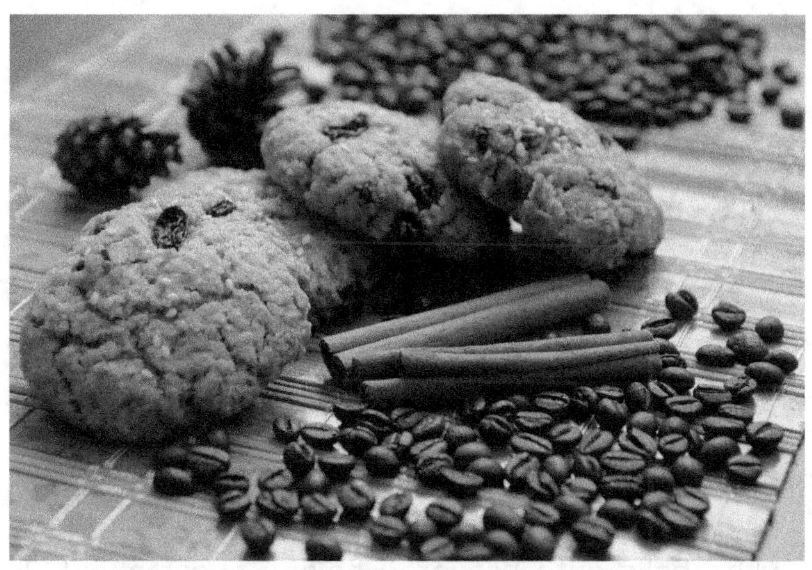

Chocolate Fat Bombs

Total time: 25 minutes

Ingredients:

8 ounces cream cheese, softened

½ cup crunchy almond butter

½ cup unsalted butter, softened

½ cup golden monk fruit sweetener

2 ounces 70% dark chocolate, finely chopped

Directions

Add the cream cheese, almond butter, butter, and monk fruit sweetener in a bowl and with an electric mixer, mix until well blended.

Transfer the mixture into refrigerator for about 30 minutes.

Remove from refrigerator and fold in the chopped chocolate.

Make 24 equal-sized balls from the mixture.

Arrange the balls onto 2 parchment-lined baking sheets in a single layer and freeze for about 45 minutes before serving.

Serve.

Mini Blueberry Bites

Total time: 25 minutes

Ingredients:

1 cup almond flour

½ cup pecans

½ cup fresh blueberries

4 ounces soft goat cheese

1 teaspoon organic vanilla extract

½ teaspoon stevia powder

¼ cup unsweetened coconut, shredded

Directions

Add the flour, pecans, blueberries, goat cheese, vanilla extract and stevia in a food processor and pulse until mixed completely.

Make 30 equal-sized balls from the mixture.

Coat the balls with shredded coconut.

Arrange the balls onto a parchment-lined baking sheet in a single layer and freeze for about 30-40 minutes before serving.

Serve.

Chocolate Coconut Bars

Total time: 28 minutes

Ingredients:

1 cup coconut oil

½ can full-fat coconut milk

½ cup desiccated coconut

1 tablespoon coconut flour

1 teaspoon organic vanilla extract

¼ cup cacao powder

¼ cup coconut oil, melted

4-5 drops liquid stevia

Directions

For coconut filling: add 1 cup of coconut oil and coconut milk in a pan over low heat and cook for about 2-3 minutes, stirring continuously.

Add the desiccated coconut and stir to combine

In the pan of coconut milk mixture, add the coconut flour, 1 tablespoon at a time and cook until the mixture resembles a porridge, beating continuously.

Remove the pan of mixture from heat and stir in vanilla extract.

Set the mixture aside to cool for about 10 minutes.

Place the coconut mixture evenly into a loaf pan and with the back of a spoon, press in 1-inch thick layer.

With a plastic wrap, cover the loaf pan and freeze for at least 5 hours or up to overnight.

Remove from the freezer and set aside at room temperature for about 20-25 minutes.

Place the cacao powder, melted coconut oil and stevia in a bowl and beat until well combined.

Cut the coconut filling into 9 equal-sized bars.

Dip each bar into the cacao powder mixture.

Arrange the bars onto a wax paper lined baking sheet and freeze until set before serving.

Serve.

Walnut Bark

Total time: 16 minutes 40 seconds

Ingredients:

For Bark:

¼ cup coconut oil

¼ cup natural peanut butter

1 teaspoon organic vanilla extract

8 drops liquid vanilla stevia

1 cup walnuts, chopped

Pinch of salt

For Chocolate Drizzle:

1 ounce 70% dark chocolate, chopped

1 teaspoon coconut oil

Directions

For bark: line 2 large plates with parchment paper.

Place the coconut oil and peanut butter in a microwave-safe bowl and microwave on High for about 30-40 seconds.

Remove the bowl from microwave and stir in the remaining ingredients.

Divide the mixture evenly onto each plate.

For drizzle: in a microwave-safe bowl, add the chocolate and coconut oil and microwave on High for about 1 minute.

Drizzle chocolate mixture over the bark and freeze for about 30 minutes or until set completely before serving.

Serve.

Almond Brittles

Total time: 25 minutes

Ingredients:

1 cup almonds

¼ cup butter

½ cup Swerve

2 teaspoons organic vanilla extract

¼ teaspoon salt

1/8 teaspoon coarse salt

Directions

Line a 9x9-inch cake pan with parchment paper.

Add the butter, Swerve, vanilla and ¼ teaspoon of salt in an 8-inch nonstick skillet over medium heat and cook until well combined, stirring continuously.

Stir in the almonds and bring to a boil, stirring continuously.

Cook for about 2-3 minutes, stirring continuously.

Remove the skillet from heat and place mixture evenly into the prepared pan.

With the back of a spoon, stir to spread the almonds and sprinkle with salt.

Set aside for about 1 hour or until cooled completely.

Break into pieces and serve.

Avocado Salsa

Total time: 25 minutes

Ingredients:

1 ripe avocado, peeled, pitted and chopped

½ cup tomato, chopped

2 tablespoons onion, chopped

2 tablespoons fresh cilantro, minced

1 tablespoon olive oil

1 tablespoon fresh lime juice

Salt and ground black pepper, as required

Directions

In a large serving bowl, add all the ingredients and gently, stir to combine.

With a plastic wrap, cover the bowl and refrigerate before serving.

Enjoy!

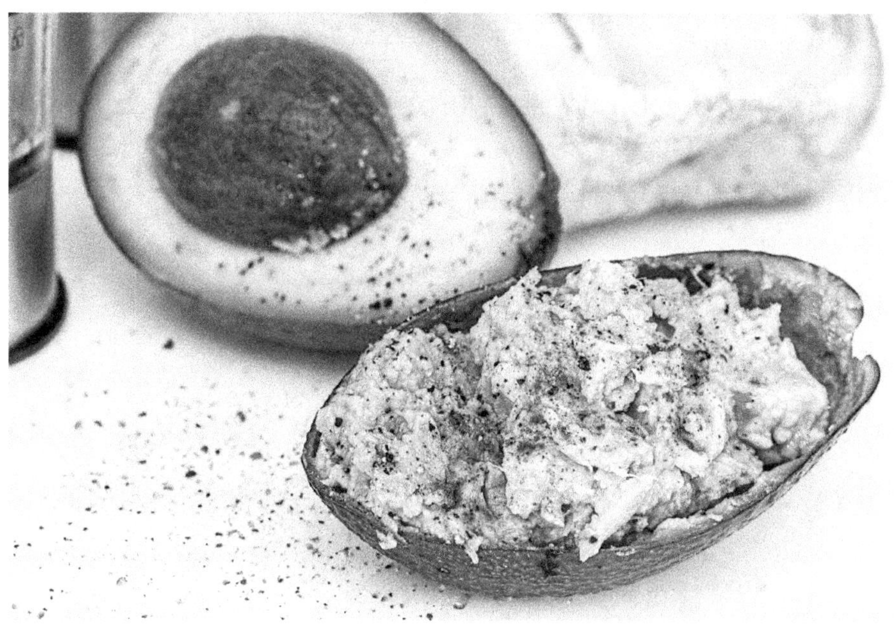

Chapter 12: Dinner Recipes

Cheese Mushroom Spinach Quiche

Total time: 55 minutes

Ingredients:

4 eggs

8 oz mushrooms, sliced

1/4 cup parmesan cheese, grated

2 oz feta cheese, crumbled

1 cup unsweetened almond milk

10 oz frozen spinach, thawed

1/2 cup mozzarella cheese, shredded

1 garlic clove, minced

Pepper

Salt

Directions:

Preheat the oven to 350 F.

Add garlic, mushrooms, pepper and salt in a pan and sauté for 5 minutes.

Greased 9-inch pie dish with cooking spray.

Add spinach in dish then places sautéed mushroom over spinach.

Sprinkle crumbled feta cheese on top.

In a bowl, whisk together eggs, parmesan cheese, and almond milk.

Pour egg mixture over spinach and mushroom then sprinkle mozzarella cheese.

Bake in oven for 45 minutes.

Slice and serve.

Zucchini Carrot Patties

Total time: 15 minutes

Ingredients:

1 egg, lightly beaten

1/2 cup carrot, grated

1 cup zucchini, grated

2 tsp coconut oil

1/3 cup mozzarella cheese, shredded

1/2 cup parmesan cheese, grated

1/4 tsp pepper

1 tsp salt

Directions:

Add all ingredients except oil into the bowl and mix until well combined.

Heat oil in a pan over medium-high heat.

Drop tablespoon of zucchini mixture on a hot pan and cook for 2 minutes on each side.

Serve and enjoy.

Tomato Zucchini Frittata

Total time: 30 minutes

Ingredients:

8 eggs

1 tbsp basil, chopped

2 tbsp olive oil

1 cup feta cheese, crumbled

1/2 cup olives, pitted and halved

1 cup grape tomatoes, cut in half

1 medium zucchini, sliced

1/2 tsp Italian seasoning

2 garlic cloves, minced

Pepper

Salt

Directions:

Heat the oven grill to medium heat.

Heat oil in a pan. Add zucchini and sauté until lightly golden.

Add garlic, Italian seasoning, and olives and cook for 1 minute.

In a bowl, whisk together eggs, pepper, and salt.

Stir in feta cheese.

Add tomatoes to a pan and pour egg mixture.

Turn heat to low and cook for 5-8 minutes.

Transfer pan to the oven and bake until frittata is set.

Garnish with basil and serve.

Italian Basil Tomato Omelet

Total time: 15 minutes

Ingredients:

2 eggs

2 oz mozzarella cheese

1 tbsp water

1 tomato, cut into thin slices

5 fresh basil leaves

1 tbsp butter

Pepper

Salt

Directions:

In a small bowl, whisk together eggs and water.

Melt butter in a pan over medium heat.

Pour egg mixture in pan and cook for 30 seconds.

Spread tomatoes, basil, and cheese on top of the omelet. Season with pepper and salt.

Cook for 2 minutes.

Serve and enjoy.

Curried Spinach

Total time: 20 minutes

Ingredients:

15 oz frozen spinach, thawed and squeeze out all liquid

2 tsp curry powder

1 tsp lemon zest

14 oz coconut milk

1/2 tsp salt

Directions:

Heat pan over medium heat.

Curry powder and few tablespoons of coconut milk and cook for a minute.

Add spinach, lemon zest, salt, and remaining milk. Stir well.

Cook spinach mixture until thickened.

Serve and enjoy.

Tofu Scramble

Total time: 20 minutes

Ingredients:

1 lb firm tofu, drained

1 cup mushrooms, sliced

1 garlic clove, minced

1 bell pepper, diced

1 tomato, diced

1 small onion, diced

Pinch of turmeric

¼ tsp onion powder

1/2 tsp pepper

1/2 tsp salt

Directions:

Heat pan over medium heat.

Add tomato, mushrooms, garlic, onion and bell pepper and sauté for 5 minutes.

Crumble tofu and add in a pan and stir with vegetables.

Add turmeric, onion powder, pepper, and salt. Stir well.

Cook for 5 minutes.

Serve and enjoy.

Cheese Herb Frittata

Total time: 3 hours 10 minutes

Ingredients:

8 eggs

4 cups baby arugula

1/2 tsp dried oregano

1/3 cup unsweetened almond milk

3/4 cup feta cheese, crumbled

1/2 cup onion, sliced

1 1/2 cups red peppers, roasted and chopped

Pepper

Salt

Directions:

Spray slow cooker with cooking spray.

In a mixing bowl, whisk eggs, oregano, and almond milk. Season with pepper and salt.

Add red peppers, onion, arugula, and cheese into the slow cooker.

Pour egg mixture over the vegetables.

Cover and cook on low for 3 hours.

Serve and enjoy.

Easy Broccoli Omelet

Total time: 20 minutes

Ingredients:

4 eggs

1 cup broccoli, chopped and cooked

1 tbsp olive oil

1 tbsp parsley, chopped

¼ tsp garlic powder

¼ tsp onion powder

1/4 tsp pepper

1/2 tsp salt

Directions:

In a bowl, whisk eggs with onion powder, garlic powder, pepper, and salt.

Heat oil in a pan over medium heat.

Pour broccoli and eggs mixture into the pan and cook until set.

Turn omelet to other side and cook until lightly golden brown.

Garnish with chopped parsley and serve.

Leek Mushroom Frittata

Total time: 45 minutes

Ingredients:

6 eggs

1 cup leeks, sliced

6 oz mushrooms, sliced

Pepper

Salt

Directions:

Preheat the oven to 350 F.

Spray pan with cooking spray and heat over medium heat.

Add mushrooms, leeks, and salt in a pan sauté for 6 minutes.

Whisk eggs in a bowl with pepper and salt.

Transfer sautéed mushroom and leek mixture into the greased baking dish.

Pour egg mixture over mushroom.

Bake in oven for 40 minutes.

Serve and enjoy.

Broccoli Cream Cheese Quiche

Total time: 150 minutes

Ingredients:

9 eggs

8 oz cream cheese

1/4 tsp onion powder

3 cups broccoli, cut into florets

2 cups cheddar cheese, shredded and divided

1/4 tsp pepper

3/4 tsp salt

Directions:

Add broccoli into the boiling water and cook for 3 minutes. Drain well and set aside to cool.

Whisk eggs, cream cheese, onion powder, pepper, and salt in mixing bowl.

Spray slow cooker with cooking spray.

Add cooked broccoli into the slow cooker then sprinkle half cup cheese.

Pour egg mixture over broccoli and cheese mixture.

Cover and cook on high for 2 hours and 15 minutes.

Sprinkle remaining cheese on top.

Cover for 10 minutes or until cheese melted.

Serve and enjoy.

Vanilla Banana Pancakes

Total time: 10 minutes

Ingredients:

2 eggs

1/8 tsp baking powder

1 large banana, mashed

2 tbsp vanilla protein powder

½ tsp vanilla

Directions:

Heat pan over medium heat.

Meanwhile, add all ingredients into the bowl and mix well until combined.

Spray pan with cooking spray.

Pour 3 tablespoons of batter onto the hot pan to make a pancake.

Cook a pancake for 30-40 seconds.

 Turn to other side and cook for 30 seconds.

Serve and enjoy.

Mozzarella Zucchini Quiche

Total time: 50 minutes

Ingredients:

3 eggs

1 cup mozzarella, shredded

15 oz ricotta

1 onion, chopped

2 medium zucchini, sliced

1/2 tsp dried oregano

1/2 tsp dried basil

1 tbsp olive oil

Pepper

Salt

Directions:

Preheat the oven to 350 F.

Sauté zucchini over low heat.

Add onion and cook for 10 minutes.

Add pepper and seasoning to zucchini mixture.

Beat eggs, and then add in mozzarella and ricotta.

Fold in onions and zucchini.

Pour egg mixture into the greased pie dish and bake in oven for 30 minutes.

Serve and enjoy.

Zucchini Breakfast Casserole

Total time: 35 minutes

Ingredients:

2 eggs

1 tbsp garlic, minced

1/2 cup onion, diced

4 cup zucchini, grated

1/2 cup cheddar cheese, shredded

1 cup mozzarella cheese, shredded

1/2 cup parmesan cheese, grated

1/2 tsp salt

Directions:

Preheat the oven to 375 F.

Add zucchini and salt into the colander and set aside for 10 minutes.

Squeeze out all liquid from zucchini.

Combine together zucchini, cheddar cheese, mozzarella cheese, 1/2 parmesan cheese, eggs, garlic, and onion and pour into the greased baking dish.

Bake in oven for 25 minutes.

Serve and enjoy.

Bacon Egg Muffins

Total time: 35 minutes

Ingredients:

12 eggs

2 tbsp fresh parsley, chopped

½ tsp mustard powder

1/3 cup heavy cream

2 green onion, chopped

4 oz cheddar cheese, shredded

8 bacon slices, cooked and crumbled

Pepper

Salt

Directions:

Preheat the oven to 375 F.

In a mixing bowl, whisk together eggs, mustard powder, heavy cream, pepper, and salt.

Divide cheddar cheese, onions, and bacon into the muffin tray cups.

Pour egg mixture into the muffin cups.

Bake in oven for 25 minutes.

Serve and enjoy.

Zucchini Ham Quiche

Total time: 50 minutes

Ingredients:

8 eggs

1 cup cheddar cheese, shredded

1 cup zucchini, shredded and squeezed

1 cup ham, cooked and diced

½ tsp dry mustard

½ cup heavy cream

Pepper

Salt

Directions:

Preheat the oven to 375 F.

Combine ham, cheddar cheese, and zucchini in a pie dish.

In a bowl, whisk together eggs, heavy cream, and seasoning. Pour egg mixture over ham mixture.

Bake in oven for 40 minutes.

Serve and enjoy.

Italian Casserole

Total time: 45 minutes

Ingredients:

2 eggs

2/3 cup parmesan cheese, grated

2/3 cup chicken broth

1 lb Italian sausage

4 egg whites

4 tsp pine nuts, minced

¼ cup roasted red pepper, sliced

¼ cup pesto sauce

1/8 tsp pepper

¼ tsp sea salt

Directions:

Preheat the oven to 400 F.

Add sausage in pan and cook until golden brown. Drain excess oil and spread it into the greased casserole dish.

Whisk remaining ingredients except pine nuts in a bowl and pour over sausage.

Bake in oven for 35 minutes.

Garnish with pine nuts and serve.

Coconut Chicken Casserole

Total time: 45 minutes

Ingredients:

2 ½ lbs chicken breasts, boneless and cubed

12 oz roasted red peppers, drained and chopped

8 garlic cloves

2/3 cup mayonnaise

5 zucchini, cut into cubes

1 tsp xanthan gum

1 tbsp tomato paste

5.4 oz coconut cream

1 tsp salt

Directions:

Preheat the oven to 400 F.

Add zucchini and chicken to a casserole dish. Cover dish with foil.

Bake in oven for 25 minutes. Stir well and cook for 10 minutes more.

Meanwhile, in a bowl, stir together remaining ingredients.

Pour bowl mixture over chicken and zucchini and broil on high for 5 minutes.

Serve and enjoy.

Healthy Carrot Noodles

Total time: 20 minutes

Ingredients:

5 medium carrots

3 garlic cloves, chopped

1/4 cup fresh spring onions, chopped

1/2 cup basil leaves

1 cup fresh parsley

3 tbsp red chili pepper flakes, crushed

2/3 cup olive oil

1/4 cup vinegar

Salt

Directions:

Add red chili flakes, oil, vinegar, garlic, spring onions, basil, and parsley in a blender and blend until smooth. Pour paste into a mixing bowl.

Add water and salt in a pot and bring to boil.

Peel carrots and using slicer make noodles.

Add carrot noodles in boiling water and blanch for 2 minutes.

Add cooked noodles in large bowl and toss well with paste.

Serve and enjoy.

Chapter 13 : Dessert Recipes

Strawberry Pancakes

Total time: 50 minutes

Ingredients:

1 cup cream cheese

5 large eggs

1/2 tbsp psyllium husk powder

1 tsp vanilla extract

1/4 cup coconut flour

2 tbsp butter

1/4 tsp salt

For the topping:

1/2 tsp stevia powder

1/2 strawberry extract

1 cup whipped cream

Directions:

In a large mixing bowl, combine coconut flour, psyllium husk powder, and salt. Mix well and then gradually add eggs. Beat with an electric mixer for 3 minutes

Now; add butter, cream cheese, and vanilla extract. Continue to beat until all well combined, Set aside

Plug in the instant pot and grease the stainless steel insert with some cooking spray. Pour about 1/3 of the mixture in the pot and close the lid. Adjust the steam release handle and press the *Manual* button. Set the timer for 3 minutes. Cook on *High* pressure

When done; perform a quick pressure release and carefully transfer to a large plate. Repeat the process with the remaining mixture

Now; prepare the topping. Combine all ingredients in a large bowl and mix until well combined. Divide the mixture evenly and top each pancake

Keto Vanilla Cherry Panna Cotta

Total time: 20 minutes

Ingredients:

For the vanilla layer:

1 cup heavy whipping cream

1/2 tsp vanilla extract

1 tbsp walnuts; roughly chopped.

2 tbsp whole milk

1 tsp agar powder

For the cherry layer:

1 tbsp almonds; roughly chopped.

2 tsp cherry extract

1 cup heavy whipping cream

1 tsp agar powder

Directions:

Plug in the instant pot and combine all vanilla layer ingredients in the stainless steel insert. Press the *Saute* button and stir constantly. Bring it to a light simmer and then press *Cancel'* button. Transfer to a large bowl and set aside

Clean the pot and pat-dry with a kitchen paper. Now; add all cherry layer ingredients and stir well. Again, bring it to a light simmer, stirring constantly

Pour about 1/2-inch thick vanilla layer in a medium-sized glass. Now; add the second layer of the cherry mixture. Repeat the process until you have used both mixtures

Optionally, garnish with some fresh mint and refrigerate for at least 1 hour before serving.

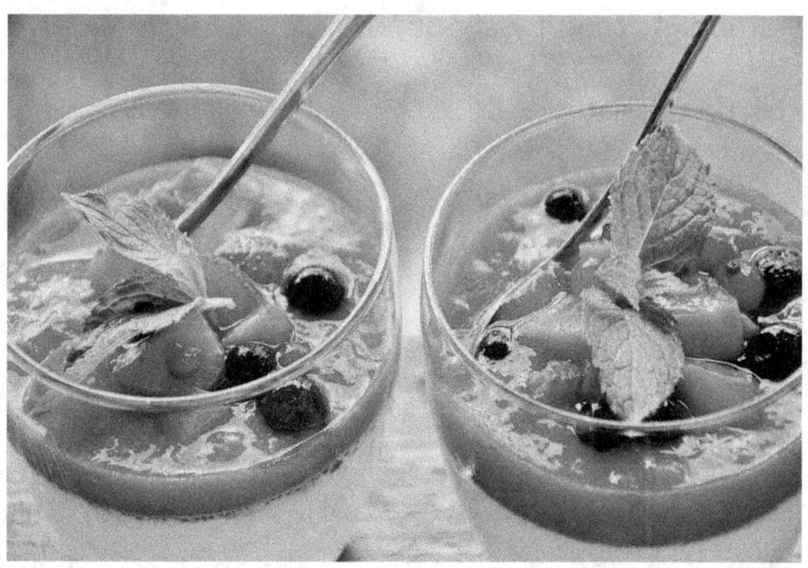

Delicious Vanilla Cream with Raspberries

Total time: 20 minutes

Ingredients:

1 ½ cup coconut milk; full-fat

1 tbsp almond flour

2 tbsp butter

1/4 cup raspberries

3 egg yolks

3 tbsp swerve

1 tbsp agar powder

1 vanilla bean

2 tsp vanilla extract

Directions:

Using a sharp paring knife, slice the vanilla bean lengthwise and remove the seeds, Set aside

Plug in the instant pot and press the *Saute* button.

Grease the inner pot with butter and add coconut milk. Warm up, stirring constantly, and then add egg yolks, swerve, and vanilla extract

Cook for 3 - 4 minutes, stirring constantly

Finally, add agar powder, and vanilla seeds. Give it a good stir and continue to cook for another couple of minutes, or until the mixture thickens.

Press the *Cancel'* button and remove the cream from the pot. Divide between serving bowls and optionally top with some whipped cream or fresh strawberries.

Plug in the instant pot and pour in the milk. Press the *Saute* button and heat up. Add swerve, cocoa powder, coconut cream, and vanilla extract.

Bring it to a boil, stirring constantly, and then add agar powder. Continue to cook for 1 - 2 minutes.

Press the *Cancel'* button and stir in finely chopped almonds.

Transfer the mixture to a large mixing bowl and pour in the whipping cream. Beat well on high speed for 2 - 3 minutes.

Finally, divide the mixture between serving bowls and top each with raspberries. Serve cold.

Keto Mocha de Creme

Total time: 30 minutes

Ingredients:

2 large eggs; separated

1 cup coconut milk; full-fat

3 tbsp brewed espresso

3 tbsp stevia powder

¾ cup heavy cream

2 tbsp cocoa powder; unsweetened

1 tsp vanilla extract

1/4 tsp salt

Directions:

In a small bowl, whisk together eggs, cocoa powder, espresso, stevia powder, vanilla, and salt, Set aside

Plug in the instant pot and press the *Saute* button. Pour in the coconut milk and heavy cream. Give it a good stir and warm up

Press the *Cancel'* button and slowly pour the warm milk mixture over the egg mixture, whisking constantly

Divide the mixture between 4 ramekins and loosely cover with aluminum foil.

Position a trivet at the bottom of your pot and pour in 2 cups of water. Gently place the ramekins on top and seal the lid

Set the steam release handle to the *Sealing* position and press the *Manual* button.

Cook for 15 minutes.

When done; perform a quick pressure release and open the lid. Remove the ramekins and transfer to a wire rack. Cool to a room temperature and then refrigerate for about an hour.

Keto Mint Brownies

Total time: 45 minutes

Ingredients:

¾ cup almond flour

2 tbsp butter

1/2 cup Mascarpone

1/2 cup flaxseed meal

4 large eggs

1/4 cup swerve

3 tbsp hazelnuts; finely chopped.

1 tsp mint extract

1/4 tsp salt

Directions:

Combine the ingredients in a large mixing bowl and beat well on medium speed until fully incorporated and smooth.

Line a small cake pan with parchment paper and brush with some oil. Pour in the batter and loosely cover with aluminum foil

Plug in the instant pot and set the trivet in the inner pot. Pour in about one cup of water and place the cake pan on top

Seal the lid and set the steam release handle to the *Sealing* position. Press the *Manual* button and set the timer for 25 minutes.

When done; perform a quick pressure release and open the lid. Carefully remove the pan from the pot and chill for a while

Slice into 8 brownies and serve

Creamy Keto Coconut Cake

Total time: 45 minutes

Ingredients:

2 cups coconut flour

1/4 cup granulated stevia

2 cups whipping cream; sugar-free

3 tsp baking powder

1 cup coconut cream

5 large eggs

3 tbsp hazelnuts; finely chopped.

1/4 cup almond flour

3 tbsp shredded coconut

2 tsp vanilla extract

Directions:

Plug in the instant pot and pour in one cup of water. Position a trivet at the bottom of the inner pot and set aside,

In a large mixing bowl, combine all dry ingredients and mix well. Add eggs, one at the time, and beat well on medium-high speed

Now add coconut cream and vanilla extract. Continue to beat for 2 more minutes on medium speed

Grease a small springform pan with some coconut oil and pour in the mixture. Place in the pot and seal the lid. Set the steam release handle and press the *Manual* button. Set the timer for 20 minutes on high pressure

Meanwhile; beat well the whipping cream until light and fluffy. Add chopped hazelnuts and optionally some finely chopped almonds

Refrigerate until use

When you hear the cooker's end signal, perform a quick pressure release and open the lid. Remove the pan from the pot and cool for a while

Top with whipped cream and refrigerate for 2 - 3 hours before serving.

Almond Vanilla Brownies

Total time: 45 minutes

Ingredients:

¾ cup almond flour

1/4 cup cocoa powder; unsweetened

1/3 cup coconut cream

1/4 cup raw almonds; finely chopped.

4 tbsp granulated stevia

2 tsp baking powder

1/4 cup flaxseed meal

3 large eggs

2 tbsp butter; melted

2 tsp vanilla extract

Directions:

In a medium-sized bowl, combine together almond flour, flaxseed meal, cocoa powder, stevia, and baking powder. Mix well and then add eggs, butter, vanilla extract, chopped almonds, and coconut cream. Using a hand mixer beat well until fully incorporated

Line a fitting cake pan with some parchment paper. Pour in the batter and shake the pan a couple of times to flatten the surface.

Seal the lid and set the steam release handle. Press the *Manual* button and cook for 25 minutes on high pressure

When done; perform a quick pressure release and open the lid. Remove the pan and cool completely before slicing.

Special Strawberry Cream Cake

Total time: 2 hours 20 minutes

Ingredients:

For the crust:

1 cup almond flour

3 tbsp swerve

1/4 cup almond butter; softened

1 cup shredded coconut

2 tsp baking powder

1 tsp baking soda

4 large eggs

1/4 tsp salt

For the cream layer:

1/4 cup swerve

1 tsp vanilla extract

6 large eggs

1/4 cup heavy cream

¾ cup cream cheese

Directions:

Plug in the instant pot and position a trivet at the bottom of the inner pot. Pour in 2 cups of water and set aside

Now prepare the crust. In a large mixing bowl, combine together all dry ingredients and mix well. Now add eggs and softened almond butter. With a dough hook on, beat until completely smooth.

Line a 6-inch springform pan with some parchment paper and pour the mixture in. flatten the surface with a kitchen spatula and set aside

In a medium-sized bowl, combine all the ingredients for the cream layer. Mix well with kitchen whisker and pour over the crust

Tightly wrap the pan with some aluminum foil and place in the pot. Seal the lid and set the steam release handle to the *Sealing* position.

Press the *Slow Cook* button and set the timer for 2 hours on low pressure

When done; perform a quick pressure release by moving the pressure valve to the *Venting* position.

Carefully open the lid and remove the cake. Cool to a room temperature and transfer to the refrigerator overnight.

Yummy Chocolate Cupcakes

Total time: 30 minutes

Ingredients:

1 ½ cups of almond flour

1/4 cup swerve

2 tbsp cocoa powder; unsweetened

1 cup shredded coconut

2 large eggs

1/4 cup cream cheese

3 tbsp butter

2 tsp baking powder

1/4 cup blueberries

3 tbsp plain Greek yogurt

1 tsp vanilla extract

Directions:

In a large mixing bowl, combine together eggs and butter. Beat well on high speed until light and fluffy mixture. Then add swerve, cream cheese, and Greek yogurt. Continue to mix until smooth.

Finally, add almond flour, shredded coconut, and baking powder. Mix well again and fold in blueberries.

Divide the mixture between 6 silicone cups and set aside

Plug in the instant pot and position a trivet at the bottom of the inner pot. Pour in 1 cup of water and carefully place cups on the trivet

Seal the lid and set the steam release handle to the *Sealing* position. Set the timer for 10 minutes on the *Manual* mode

Perform a quick pressure release and open the lid. Remove the cups from the pot and cool to a room temperature

Coconut Flan

Total time: 39 minutes

Ingredients:

2 tablespoons water

1 cup unsweetened coconut milk

3 large eggs

Pinch salt

1 cup heavy cream

¾ cup powdered erythritol, divided

2 teaspoons vanilla extract

Directions:

Whisk together ½ cup of the powdered erythritol and water in a saucepan over medium heat until it starts to darken. Divide the mixture among six small ramekins and set aside to cool.

Combine the coconut milk and cream in a saucepan and cook over medium heat until it starts to steam then whisk in the rest of the erythritol and the vanilla extract. Beat the eggs in a mixing bowl then pour a few tablespoons of the warmed milk into it while whisking.

Pour the egg mixture into the milk mixture and whisk smooth then pour into the ramekins.

Cover the ramekins with foil and place them in the steamer insert in your Instant Pot. Pour in ½ cup water then close and lock the lid.

Press the Manual button and adjust the timer for 9 minutes.

When the timer goes off, let the pressure vent naturally then press Cancel.

When the pot has depressurized, open the lid.

Remove the ramekins and let the flan cool to room temperature then chill until ready to serve.

Blueberry Mug Cake

Total time: 25 minutes

Ingredients:

4 large eggs

¼ cup sugar-free maple syrup

1 1/3 cup almond flour

½ cup fresh blueberries

¼ teaspoon salt

2 teaspoons vanilla extract

Directions:

Place the trivet in the Instant Pot and add 1 cup of water.

Whisk together the almond flour, egg, sugar-free maple syrup, vanilla, and salt in a mixing bowl.

Fold in the blueberries then divide the mixture among four 8-ounce jars.

Cover the jars with foil then place on the trivet, close and lock the lid.

Press the Manual button and adjust the timer to 10 minutes.

When the timer goes off, do a Quick Release by pressing Cancel and switching the steam valve to "venting".

When the pot has depressurized, open the lid.

Remove the jars and let them cool a little before serving.

Ricotta Lemon Cheesecake

Total time: 45 minutes

Ingredients:

1/3 cup whole-milk ricotta cheese

2 large eggs

1 (8-ouncepackage cream cheese, softened

¼ cup powdered erythritol

Juice and zest of 1 lemon

½ teaspoon lemon extract

Directions:

Combine all of the ingredients except the eggs in a mixing bowl.

Beat until the mixture is smooth then adjust sweetener to taste.

Lower the mixer speed and blend in the eggs until they are fully incorporated, being careful not to overmix.

Grease a 6-inch springform pan and pour in the cheesecake mixture.

Cover the pan with foil and place it in the Instant Pot on top of the trivet.

Pour in 2 cups of water then close and lock the lid.

Press the Manual button and adjust the timer for 30 minutes on High Pressure.

When the timer goes off, let the pressure vent naturally.

When the pot has depressurized, open the lid.

Let the cheesecake cool a little then chill for at least 8 hours before serving.

Creamy Lemon Curd

Total time: 30 minutes

Ingredients:

2 large eggs

2 large egg yolks

3 ounces butter

2/3 cup lemon juice

1 cup powdered erythritol

Directions:

Combine the butter and erythritol in a mixing bowl and beat for 2 minutes.

Whisk together the eggs and yolks then drizzle them into the bowl while mixing.

Add the lemon juice and mix until well combined.

Divide the mixture among three half-pint jars and loosely cover with the lids.

Place the jars in the Instant Pot on the trivet then pour in 1 ½ cups water.

Close and lock the lid.

Press the Manual button and adjust the timer to 10 minutes on High Pressure.

When the timer goes off, let the pressure vent for 10 minutes then do a Quick Release by pressing Cancel and switching the steam valve to "venting".

When the pot has depressurized, open the lid.

Let the curd thicken for 20 minutes at room temperature then chill.

Chocolate Pudding Cake

Total time: 24 minutes

Ingredients:

2/3 cup stevia-sweetened dark chocolate

½ cup unsweetened applesauce

2 large eggs

½ cup almond flour

1 teaspoon vanilla extract

¼ cup unsweetened cocoa powder

Directions:

Melt the chocolate in a double boiler over low heat until melted.

In a mixing bowl, whisk together the applesauce, eggs, and vanilla extract.

Whisk in the almond flour and cocoa powder then stir in the melted chocolate.

Pour the mixture into a greased 6-inch cake pan.

Place the pan in the Instant Pot on top of the trivet and pour in 2 cups of water.

Close and lock the lid.

Press the Manual button and adjust the timer on High Pressure for 4 minutes.

When the timer goes off, do a Quick Release by pressing Cancel and switching the steam valve to "venting".

When the pot has depressurized, open the lid.

Remove the pan and let the cake cool 10 minutes before removing.

Mini Vanilla Custards

Total time: 39 minutes

Ingredients:

2 tablespoons water

1 cup unsweetened almond milk

3 large eggs

Pinch salt

1 cup heavy cream

¾ cup powdered erythritol, divided

1 tablespoon vanilla extract

Directions:

Whisk together ½ cup of the powdered erythritol and water in a saucepan over medium heat until the erythritol melts.

Divide the mixture among four small ramekins and set aside to cool.

Combine the almond milk and cream in a saucepan and cook over medium heat until it starts to steam then whisk in the rest of the erythritol and the vanilla extract.

Beat the eggs in a mixing bowl.

Whisk a few tablespoons of the milk mixture into the eggs then whisk in the rest in a steady stream.

Cover the ramekins with foil and place them in the steamer insert in your Instant Pot.

Pour in ½ cup water then close and lock the lid.

Press the Manual button and adjust the timer for 9 minutes.

When the timer goes off, let the pressure vent naturally then press Cancel.

When the pot has depressurized, open the lid.

Remove the ramekins and let the custards cool for 10 minutes then serve warm.

Coconut Almond Cake

Total time: 55 minutes

Ingredients:

½ cup unsweetened shredded coconut

2 large eggs

½ cup heavy cream

¼ cup butter, melted

1 cup almond flour

6 tablespoons powdered erythritol

1 teaspoon baking powder

Directions:

Whisk together the almond flour, coconut, erythritol, and baking powder in a mixing bowl.

Add the eggs, heavy cream, and butter then whisk smooth.

Pour into a greased 6-inch cake pan and cover with foil.

Place the steamer rack in the Instant Pot and add 2 cups of water.

Put the cake pan on the steamer rack then close and lock the lid.

Press the Manual button and adjust the timer to 40 minutes at High Pressure.

When the timer goes off, let the pressure vent for 10 minutes then do a Quick Release by pressing Cancel and switching the steam valve to "venting".

When the pot has depressurized, open the lid.

Remove the cake and let it cool in the pan for 15 minutes before turning out.

Maple Almond Cake in a Jar

Total time: 25 minutes

Ingredients:

3 large eggs

¼ teaspoon salt

1 cup almond flour

1 ½ teaspoons vanilla extract

3 tablespoons sugar-free maple syrup

Directions:

Place the trivet in the Instant Pot and add 1 cup of water.

Whisk together the almond flour, egg, sugar-free maple syrup, vanilla, and salt in a mixing bowl.

Divide the mixture among three 8-ounce jars.

Cover the jars with foil then place on the trivet, close and lock the lid.

Press the Manual button and adjust the timer to 10 minutes.

When the timer goes off, do a Quick Release by pressing Cancel and switching the steam valve to "venting".

When the pot has depressurized, open the lid.

Remove the jars and let them cool a little before serving.

Easy Chocolate Cheesecake

Total time: 50 minutes

Ingredients:

1/3 cup whole-milk ricotta cheese

2 large eggs

1 (8-ouncepackage cream cheese, softened

¼ cup powdered erythritol

1 teaspoon vanilla extract

¼ cup unsweetened cocoa powder

Directions:

Combine all of the ingredients except the eggs in a mixing bowl.

Beat until the mixture is smooth then adjust sweetener to taste.

Lower the mixer speed and blend in the eggs until they are fully incorporated, being careful not to overmix.

Grease a 6-inch springform pan and pour in the cheesecake mixture.

Cover the pan with foil and place it in the Instant Pot on top of the trivet.

Pour in 2 cups of water then close and lock the lid.

Press the Manual button and adjust the timer for 30 minutes on High Pressure.

When the timer goes off, let the pressure vent naturally.

When the pot has depressurized, open the lid.

Let the cheesecake cool a little then chill for at least 6 hours before serving.

Classic Crème Brulee

Total time: 24 minutes

Ingredients:

6 large egg yolks

2 tablespoons granular erythritol

2 cups heavy cream

3 tablespoons powdered erythritol

1 tablespoon vanilla extract

Directions:

Whisk together the heavy cream, egg yolks, powdered erythritol, and the vanilla in a bowl.

Divide the mixture among 6 small ramekins and cover with foil.

Place the steamer rack in the Instant Pot and add 1 cup water.

Place the ramekins in the steamer rack, offsetting the stacks so they are stable.

Close and lock the lid then press the Manual button and adjust the timer to 9 minutes.

When the timer goes off, let the pressure vent for 15 minutes then do a Quick Release by pressing Cancel and switching the steam valve to "venting".

When the pot has depressurized, open the lid.

Remove the ramekins and chill until they are cold.

Sprinkle the granular erythritol over the crème brulees and place under the broiler until browned.

Let the topping harden before serving.

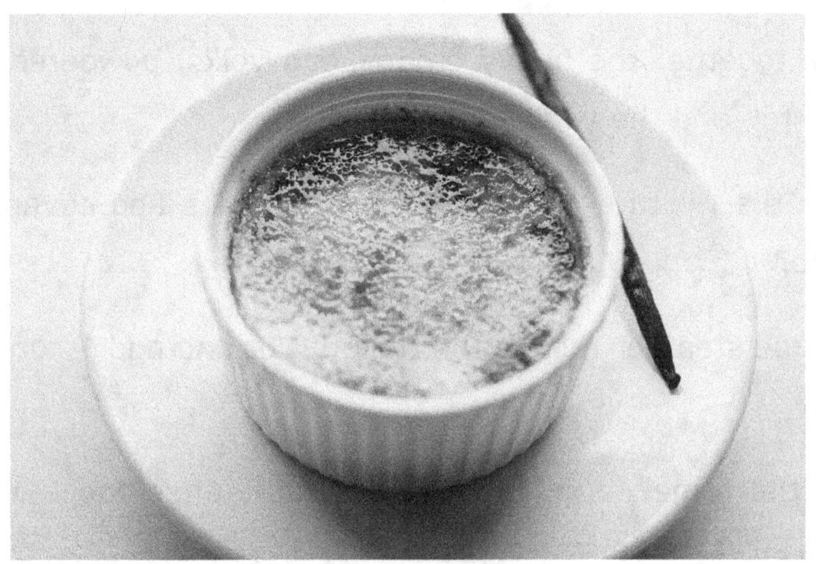

Chili Cauliflower Spread

Total time: 30 minutes

Ingredients:

1 (choppedShallot

1 pound Cauliflower florets

¼ cup Chicken stock

2 (choppedRed hot chilies

2 tbsp (mincedGinger

1 tbsp Avocado oil

1 and ¼ tbsp Balsamic vinegar

Directions:

Let your Instant Pot preheat on Sauté mode.

Add oil, ginger, and scallions, then sauté for 2 minutes.

Stir in remaining ingredients and mix well

Seal the pot's lid and cook for 13 minutes on manual mode at High.

Allow the pressure to release in 10 minutes naturally then remove the lid.

Blend the mixture with a hand held blender until smooth.

Serve fresh and enjoy.

CONCLUSION

Thanks for making it through to the end of this book, we hope it was informative and able to provide you with all of the tools you need to achieve your goals, whatever it is that they may be. Just because you've finished this book doesn't mean there is nothing left to learn on the topic, and expanding your horizons is the only way to find the mastery you seek.

Now that you have made it to the end of this book, you hopefully have an understanding of how to get started with the keto diet, as well as a strategy or two, or three, that you are anxious to try for the first time. Before you go ahead and start giving it your all, however, it is important that you have realistic expectations as to the level of success you should expect in the near future.

While it is perfectly true that some people experience serious success right out of the gate, it is an unfortunate fact of life that they are the exception rather than the rule. What this means is that you should expect to experience something of a learning curve, especially when you are first figuring out what works for you. This is perfectly normal, however, and if you persevere you will come out the other side better because of it. Instead of getting your hopes up to an unrealistic degree, you should think of your time spent maximizing your weight loss as a marathon rather than a sprint which means that slow and steady will win the race every single time.

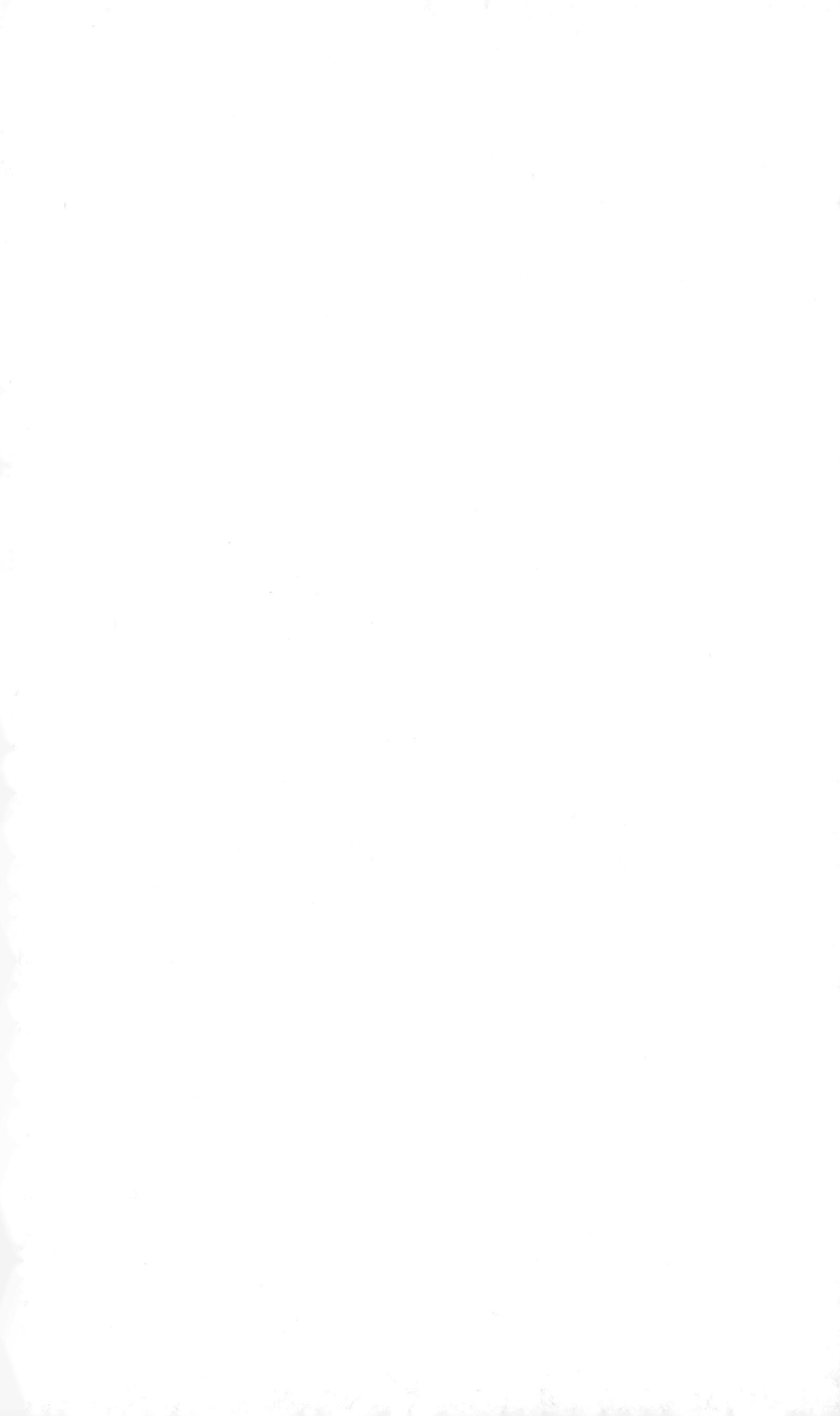

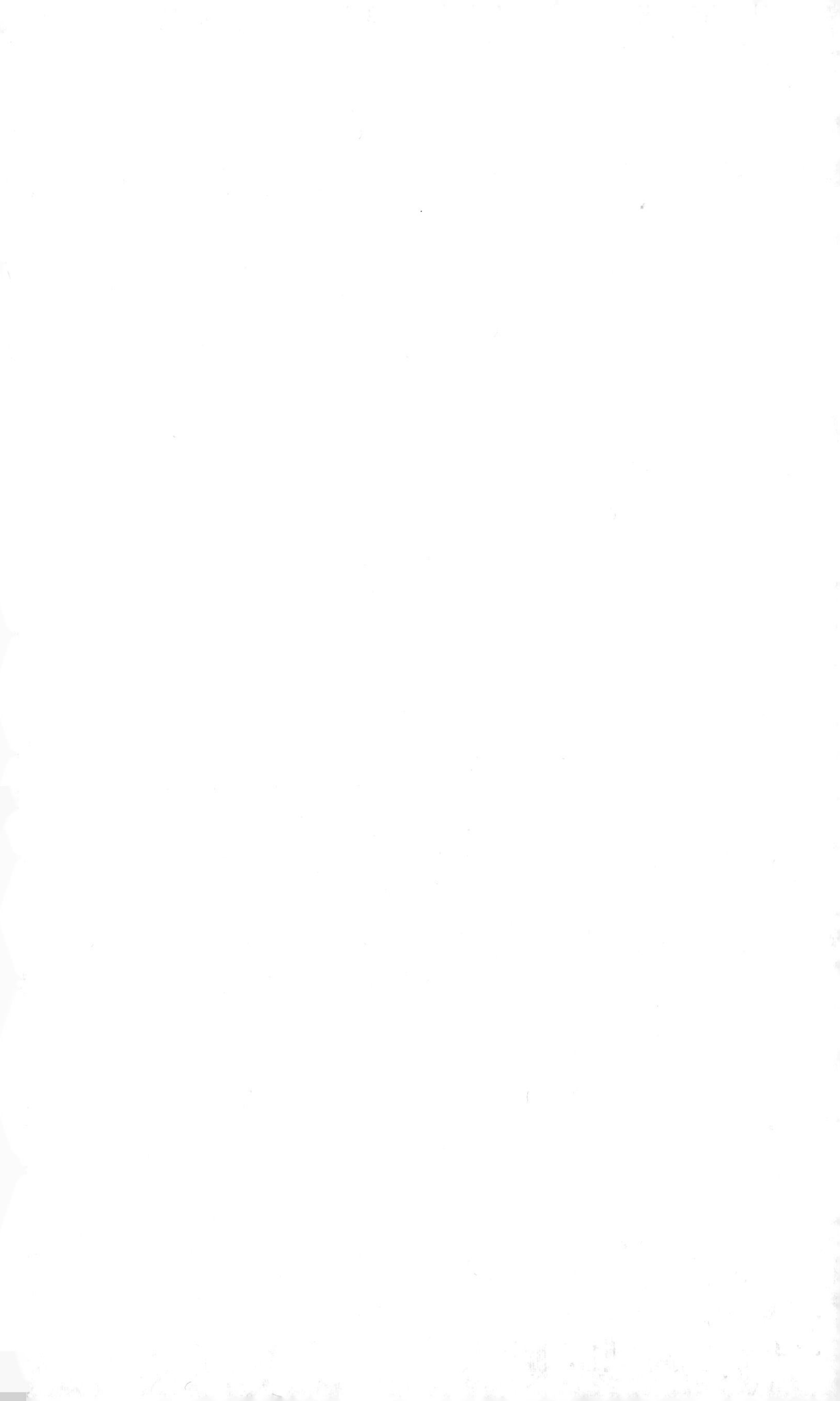

www.ingramcontent.com/pod-product-compliance
Lightning Source LLC
Chambersburg PA
CBHW070652250726
48662CB00001B/79